MW00437103

YOUR TEMPLE

Holistic Health & Healing

A guide for a Better Body and Optimal Health

Dr. Angie Cross, D.C.

ISBN-10:0615687520

ISBN-13: 978-0615687520 (Dr. Angie Cross, D.C.)

CONTENTS

DEDICATION

I would like to dedicate this book to all my patients who have not given up hope. I would like this to be a guide to inspire you to keep on keeping on. I would like to also dedicate this to book to all the people looking for a new beginning in their life.

ACKNOWLEDGMENTS

There are so many people who have inspired me along this journey and so many people who work behind the scenes on all my many projects. I often times assume these people know how important they are to me. However, I would like to take a moment to express my heart felt, sincere thanks and gratitude towards those people who have been a blessing to me and my life. I want to let them know how grateful I am that our paths have crossed during this journey.

My first big thank you goes out to God our Father and his Son Jesus Christ. Without God in my life, I am nothing. I am here to be his servant. He has put the love for health and the desire to help people deep within my soul. Thank you for making me the woman that I am today. I want to thank him for always loving us, no matter what. Our bodies are called our "Temples" in the bible and God has allowed me to be a teacher to the world on how we can best care for our "Temples".

After God, my first big hug goes out to my favorite person in the world, my mom! You have been there for me through all the "adventures", both good and bad. You have always been supportive, encouraging, and so very loving. I am truly blessed to have you in my corner. I am blessed that God chose you to be my mom. I will forever be grateful for you mom!

Second on my list to thank is my dad. I love you dad for loving mom so much. I love you for instilling family values into me. I love you for some "tough love" that I very much needed along my journey. You have been there, along with mom, through my fun "adventures". You have always believed in me and been supportive towards my decisions in life. Thank you Dad!

A big special mommy hug goes out to my two little loves of my life, Stryker and Olivia. You are the reason I strive to be the best I can be every day. You both are my pride and joy. You both have such incredible attitudes towards life and to love and serve. You will both grow up to make a positive difference in the world. I love you so much!

I offer a big thank you and a huge hug to Bobby Jones. You have inspired me on so many levels. The project of writing this book has been in thought for years, but you encouraged me to put it into action. You have been there for the entire process. Thank you for your many prayers, time, support, encouragement, and friendship. Thank you for your openness to talk about life, love, pressures of the world and encouragement in trusting the Lord. Thank you for helping me become a better woman through the many hours of Bible study and discussion on spirituality and always reminding me to have a "RMA". Thank you for opening up a side of me that I am so amazed with. Thank you for the many special moments of art and creativity filled with joy. I have enjoyed the many adventures we have taken. You mean the world to me.

A special thank you for my friend Stephanie Fisher, a nutritional health and wellness coach, who helped me format and edit the book. The many hours you contributed to this project will forever be appreciated more than words can say. Your wisdom and passion for the topic of health and nutrition is priceless. You are an asset to the world of health and healing.

A big hug goes out to my niece Sydnie Pottebaum. You were such a big help in so many ways. The many hours you helped with pulling pieces together are much appreciated. I look forward to our future projects.

My dear friend Wendy Bakke, you are a gem. Your support and patience with me to complete this project will not go unforgotten. You went above and beyond to keep our YOLI team going while pulling this project through to completion. You are an amazing woman and I have enjoyed the journey over the last year and look forward to the future.

My lifelong friend, Stacie Feilmeier, you have been my supporter, encourager, and cheerleader in all areas of my life. You have seen me grow, cry, laugh, become a mom, and been there through all my adventures of life. You have kept me on track and held my hand many times. Thank you from the bottom of my heart. You mean so much to me, more than words could ever express.

Dr. Teri Cooper, You made more of an impact on me than you will ever realize. You taught me many amazing steps in becoming an alternative holistic healer. You inspired me to do acupuncture, herbs, detoxing, emotional work, and all the "fun stuff". You inspire so many people every day. You are a wonderful woman in the world of alternative healing.

To my office staff over the last ten years, especially Shari, Julie, Julie, Bobby Jo, Jan, Mikayla, and Sharlene. You all have been my support, helpers, and advocates for natural health and healing. I personally want to thank each one of you for believing and supporting my message. I want to thank you for your patience with all of my adventures, trials, tribulations and projects.

I know it couldn't be easy some days, but you always showed up with smiles, an attitude to serve patients, and always went above and beyond your job duties. Thank you so much.

My friend, Renee Wittrock, over the years you have inspired me to get my message out there. You were the one who first mentioned I should write a book. Thank you for your friendship, business ideas, support, and encouragement over all the years. All the "visualizing" moments set all this into motion. Exciting to see where things are for both of us now.

To all other family and friends, huge hugs and thank you from the bottom of my heart for your support, encouragement, and love over the years. It has been an adventure to say the least on this journey. You have all been such amazing "God winks" in my life. Thank you.

To my mentor, Dr. Jack Donovan, You have encouraged me, supported me, and taught me along the way. Your wisdom and presence speaks nothing but Health and Healing. Your love for chiropractic impresses me every time I am near you. Thank you for who you are, all you stand for, and your solid love for life.

To my mentor Dr. John Brimhall, you amaze me. You are always thinking of ways to improve the healing world. You are an inspiration to me with how you pulled the different steps to wellness all together in an easy to use system. Thank you.

To DD and BJ Palmer, The men who were brilliant enough to bring chiropractic to the world. I am amazed at the brilliance of "the art, science, and philosophy of chiropractic". Without these two men, the world of natural healing would not be where it is today. This profession has saved millions of people from unnecessary drugs and surgeries every year. What a testimony to the human body at its finest.

And finally, to all the people I have worked with over the years. The people who lost hope and found it again. The people who searched for second opinions and believed in my words. The people who were ready to give up and they gave it one more chance. Thank you for believing in holistic health and healing avenues. Thank you for your time, support, and belief in me as your health provider. You all amaze me. I am always in complete "awe" of the human soul. I have learned so much about the human soul, the strength people have and the determination you need to keep fighting the battles. What an amazing journey this has been, I feel so privileged to serve God through the gift of healing and teaching.

Chapter 1

Opposing Views on Health

"Your body is a temple of the HOLY SPIRIT, who is in you, whom you have received from God. You are not your own; you were bought at a price therefore honor God with your bodies." 1 Corinthians 6:19-20

Philosophy, we all have one on health whether you realize it or not. We all have our beliefs, thoughts, and philosophical views. Who really holds the right answer? It all depends on what views you have been exposed to, other people's opinions, and what you have been taught about health and disease. Your philosophy may depend on what part of country you live in. It also depends on your upbringing. And most importantly, what part of the world you were born in. It is all perceptions or deceptions. I have spent a decade of unraveling the web of what people perceive as truth when it comes to health. What health is to one person is the complete opposite to another. What health means to one doctor is far opposite of what it means to a different doctor. When one doctor may run a certain test, it may be the last test a different doctor would run. What one parent would bring their child to the doctor for would be the silliest thing for a different parent bring their child to the doctors for. What one person takes for the common cold is the last thing another person may take.

The last ten years has been a complete eye opening experience on sharing moments with many other wonderful people. People want answers. People are searching for the truth. People deserve answers. The people I work with have good hearts. These people are just like you and I. These people are on the search for second opinions. They are on a quest for answers to resolve their health conditions. Many times they are left with no hope. They are left feeling helpless. Not even to be told there are alternative options. Holistic options to help heal their fatigue, headaches, digestion problems, depression, or any other variety of health issue. These beautiful souls, theses loving mothers, kind men, and innocent children are being suppressed from the truth.

Answers do exist. And many at that. There are many different ways to look at one problem. There is always a "plan B". Don't settle for a "diagnosis". That is just a label. You are a human being with a heart, with a soul, and you deserve some choices. There are many different ways to look at things. Don't give up hope. Many times you just haven't been exposed to the "other way" yet. Many times you haven't been given the alternative options to your conditions. You deserve to be educated on health. You are about to be educated on holistic health view points and certain steps to take towards health and healing.

Many times I feel like a human detective. Don't give up looking and searching for answers. I will show you some different possible causes for your conditions. This approach may not be comfortable to all people. There truly are no guarantees, but many times some basic knowledge and looking at things differently will work faster and better than drugs, surgery, or "hoping it will go away". It always made sense to me to look for the cause of problems, rather than cover it up in hopes it will go away. We need to work together. You must be teachable and open to learning new approaches on health. I will be your coach. I will pass along what I have studied, learned, witnessed, and spent thousands of hours and years dissecting to bring to you. My hope for you is to find the answers you have been searching for in this book.

The thousands of patients I have had the privilege of helping over the years has made my heart want to reach out to the world. I want people to know there are answers. You have choices. You can have vitality and health. Let me teach you. Let's put all the pieces of the puzzle together.

Many times traditional medical doctors are so busy. They are doing the best they can keeping up with insurance, overbooked schedules, ordering test, interpreting tests, learning about the newest drugs and treating the latest "common cold". They are wonderful men and women who have families and good intentions. It's not on the forefront of their minds to sit down and educate you on diet, stress, hormones, nutritional supplements or detoxification programs. They are well versed in drugs, testing, and protocol checklists. They believe medicine is the answer. They believe running you through all tests are the answers. I by no means am saying I would never visit a traditional medical doctor. There is a time and a place for each style of doctor. Just realize, many times they have to cover their mind on malpractice insurance protocols. Other times, as sad as it may sound, it may be a numbers game, "burn-out", or they are stuck in their old ways of thinking.

In the meantime, a common headache can be resolved from a chiropractic adjustment or acupuncture. Or bio-identical hormone replacement can help alleviate depression or fatigue. Finding a food allergy for an unresolved digestion problem may be an answer. Or better yet, starting magnesium and losing 15 pounds could reduce your high blood pressure. How about a pineapple enzyme called bromelain to help with inflammation. Or vitamin D for seasonal depression or increasing your energy during winter months. Did you realize cruciferous vegetables, such as broccoli and cauliflower will help reduce breast cancer risks? Or taking a hot bath with Epsom salts and baking soda can help alkalize your body, thus reducing pain and soreness.

It makes sense that our God knew what He was doing when he created us. He knew the foods that would heal our bodies. He knew that we needed time to relax and decompress. How amazing he also knew good restful sleep was our time to regenerate our cells. Or a good healthy robust sex drive was normal for a husband and wife to enjoy. God knew what he was doing. The human species is part of the ecosystem, just like the animals, plants, and soil. We are simple creatures. We operate relatively simple; the modern society has come and interfered with God's original plan.

I find it disturbing how little people know about health, their own bodies, or some natural healing remedies. We now need medications to put people to sleep. We need caffeine to get going. People sit for 8 hours in front of a glaring electronic machine, called a computer, and think it somehow doesn't affect our cells. We eat genetically modified foods. We eat foods where live enzymes have been depleted. People have lost the drive to be active. We have lost the drive to rest and relax. Society has now come to the time where we feel "guilty" if we are not doing "something". We feel lost if our smart phones are not within reach. We feel depressed if we have not stayed plugged into social media. Our children no longer know how to entertain themselves with simple things, many need electronic gadgets. Families eat drive through, pick up, microwave, boxed, frozen or takeout meals.

Now more than ever we need answers. We need to regain control of our own health. We need to take responsibility. Insurance premiums continue to rise because people are not willing to take full responsibility with action steps towards health and wellness. They 'wait and hope' it won't happen to them. They wait and see what will happen. They take medication after medication hoping their infection goes away. In the mean time they should be educated how 3 soda pops day, bad foods, and lack of sleep could be contributing to the lack of real healing. People need solutions. We need to educate America and our future to stop the insane disease epidemics and drug sales soaring out of control.

Interferences with Health

If there has been an interruption in normal physiology, health starts to deteriorate and the body functions less than one hundred percent. Once there is an interruption, chaos on some level, biochemically or structurally that has taken place. The intensity, frequency and duration of the interference will dictate the length of recovery time.

People often doubt that they can recover or overcome a major disease or condition due to our westernized medical philosophy. We have stripped people from HOPE. People have lost respect for the power of their own living temple. We have become a society so dependent on drugs, medication, and rounds of testing; to many times left to be disappointed with little answers.

Possible interferences are diet, food, stress, lack of sleep, nerve impingements of spinal nerves, medications, lifestyle, sugar, alcohol, air pollution, chemicals and toxins, over exertion, injuries, repetitive movements, old injuries, negative thought patterns, and consistent poor decision. These are a few possible interferences to optimal health and longevity.

Problems Need Fixing

I know there is something majorly wrong with our health "care" industry as recently I sat down with a new female patient who had been newly diagnosed with breast cancer and not one person asked her how her diet has been. Not one doctor or nurse has asked how much stress she has had in her life. Nobody tested her hormones, since after all she is 50 years old, going through menopause. How was her sleep? How was her water intake? How much soda does she consume? How much real food does she eat versus processed chemically filled foods? How often is she using a microwave? How much sugar is she taking in daily? Are any of these questions being asked to this helpless scared woman? NO!

This is a disgrace to the human soul trying to find answers on why her body is turning against her. She was uninformed, yet hungry for knowledge. She wanted to be educated.

Why didn't the doctors ask her these BASIC lifestyle questions? Maybe because it takes too much time. It may be due to forgetting the fundamentals of the age and menopausal year she is going through. Maybe it would require more staff? How would they start incorporating all these real lifestyle factors in to the equation? It's a new thought. It would require a change to the entire system. It's too easy. It may actually prolong and save more lives. It may actually put some health care providers out of jobs as it would actually prevent diseases in the first place.

A new branch of healthcare that should be an active part in patient care should be "patient advocates". They would be asking the very basic lifestyle, age, stress and diet related questions. Then it is up to the doctor to factor in the answers with the equation of care. It is up to the doctor or nurse to educate on diet and lifestyle habits and how it will affect the patient's outcome.

Prevention is the Key to Heath

If we would focus on ways to prevent diseases and conditions rather than treat after the fact, we could most likely get our government out of debt within a few short years. Health care costs are the leading expenses at more than $8,000.00 per person per year. (OECD, 2010) We spend 33% of the GDP on health "care" costs each year. Can we say "Houston we have a problem".

The purpose of this book is to bring awareness to you and offer some holistic views on health and healing. This is your blueprint on how to care for your precious YOUR TEMPLE, aka body, to live a long, healthy, abundant life. I have laid out specific information in each chapter as a guide towards your BETTER BODY. This guide is a way to gain a better body for you and your family to enjoy. This is new way to look at health and wellness that will save you money now and in your future. It is a way to keep aging parents out of nursing homes longer. As well as a way to keep your body in prime active mode. A step by step system to follow to keep your blood sugar stable. A program to follow to alkalize your body pH. A guide to recommendations for transitioning your thought life. If you follow the suggestions in this book you will yield your BETTER BODY. I promise something will change for the better. Enjoy the journey of learning new views.

Chapter 2

A Nation Out of Control with the "Traditional" View on "Health" Care

Health expenditures in the United States neared $2.6 trillion in 2010, over ten times the $256 billion spent in 1980. (Centers for Medicare and Medicaid Services, 2012)

What is Driving Health Care Spending?

While there is broad agreement that the rise in costs must be controlled, there is disagreement over the driving factors. The amount of pharmaceutical drugs being prescribed every year is growing exponentially each year. Yes, in 2011, doctors wrote 4.02 billion prescriptions for drugs in America. That's an average of roughly 13 prescriptions for each man, woman, and child. The cost of drugs is causing a drain in our economy faster than we can come up with a solution. I believe there is a solution to this problem: Prevention and education!!

Our society cannot handle the burden of the excessive spending on preventable diseases. We must fight for our financial and physical freedom. We need to demand changes be made. We need to demand doctors to educate people on healthy diet, stress management and exercise, rather than giving them drugs and sending them on their way, only to go home and eat fattening foods and get "numb" from their new drug. We must demand our children are being fed "real" foods in school. We must demand our senior citizens are given healthy foods and encouraged to stay active, rather than being told to buy frozen preservative filled foods and put on drugs for their aches and pains.

People need to know that simple hydration can help their physical pains to subside. They need to understand magnesium and calcium can help with depression and high blood pressure. They need to know there are hormones and antibiotics most likely added to their chicken and beef they are eating daily, only to wonder why they have major hormone problems or worse yet, cancer.

Research has shown that if people would lose just 5 percent of the average BMI (body max index) by 2030, we could save our country billions of dollars in health care costs and save millions of lives. We need to educate people. You are taking the first step in solving the catastrophic epidemic problem that has grown out of control. As a doctor, I thank you for being proactive rather than reactive. You are ten steps ahead of the game!!

I recently saw a quote stating out of 100 people: "5% make it happen, 45% watch it happen, 50% didn't even know something was happening." I will say you must be the 5% if you are reading this book and take even a few of the recommendations and take action, you will yield an improved health report card within 90 days.

More Hidden Reasons the Problems are Out of Control

The foods today have become devoid of live ingredients. Foods in the stores are stripped of the live active healthy part of the food, so they can withstand the shipping, storage, shelf life for up to two years. And we feed our bodies this 'dead' "food" and expect to feel good? We need to look at things face value and be honest with ourselves with what we are putting in our bodies.

Today there are so many hidden culprits allowing you to not feel your best. It is the man-made chemicals, additives, and food processing techniques that are the main issues. The man-made Trans fats, high fructose corn syrup, artificial sweeteners, genetically modified food, pasteurization of food, microwaving of food, growth hormones and drugs in the meat and dairy products. The "xeno-hormones" (fake hormone mimickers) found in beauty products, detergents, laundry dryer sheets, nail polish, perfumes, lotions and creams we put on our skin. Chlorine and fluoride are halogens which are known to be dangerous and toxic to the body if exposed to high levels. The water we drink and shower in are hidden culprits to the health and obesity problems of today.

A Harvard School of Public Health Study found that women who ate fast food more than twice per week had an 86% increase in their risk of being overweight.

People are on auto-pilot. So many people are just surviving. They are numb to what is going on in the hectic life. They are in denial how bad their life or health has gotten. They eat without thinking of what they are eating. They mindlessly drink their "energy" drinks filled with artificial colors, stimulants, and enough unregulated caffeine that it could give a child a heart attack.

The foods children are fed in the schools today are many times as unnatural and preservative filled as something that could last months without spoiling. Chocolate milk with 40 grams of sugar given to kids in grade school and wondering why there is a lack of attention in the class room. Do we really have to go back to school and explain that high sugar intake will indeed cause a surge in excess energy? It's basic cause and effects taking place.

People are lacking of digestive enzymes, and are nutritionally deficient, and hormonally imbalanced. Women are loading up on artificial sweeteners in 'sugar free' or 'diet' sodas, jello, yogurts, cookies, foods, and drinks thinking they are being healthy. This is how much women have been deceived by our food industry. If you do the research, aspartame, sucralose, and sugar free sweeteners are known to be excitatory neurotoxins. This means it could kill your neurons, your brain cells, and neurological tissues. Do the research, it is out there.

The reason these foods can get away with this is because technically you can put a "certain amount" in each individual food or drink product. But what is the damaging effect is the accumulative effect. It's a little here, a little there, and soon is where you will find the problem. One of the most reported substances to the FDA with negative side effects is aspartame.

Be Aware

The health problems aspartame can cause are headaches, digestive problems, numbness, vision problems, mental issues, attention issues, cardiovascular and heart irregularities. Be an educated consumer. Some of the products you can find this ingredient in are most chewing gums, diet sodas, sugar free jello, sugar free frostings, most low calorie yogurts, most low calorie prepackaged foods, certain protein shakes, or any other 'diet' product.

Never assume foods or drinks to be safe today. The industry is hungry for the bottom dollar. This is your health and your future we are talking about.

I want to teach you how to eat, when to eat, and what to eat so you don't have to count calories, eat certain foods and eliminate others, count fat or carbohydrate grams is completely unnatural and unnecessary. The rest of the world is not experiencing the problems America is. They don't have the schedules we do. They don't consume artificial foods like we do. They are not overmedicated. They take more vacations and more time to relax. We need to get control back in our country. Truly make it the land of the free. We are an educated country, lets act like it. Our health numbers are an embarrassment compared to the rest of the world.

The food is produced differently than in America. In America, for example, many times beef is injected with bovine growth hormone and loaded with antibiotics and other drugs. The grains and many foods are now genetically modified. The beef produced in America is different from the beef produced in other countries. It's not that beef makes you fat; it's the chemicals and growth hormones and drugs put in the American beef that is horrible for your health and your body.

Prepackaged food diets are one of the worst. They are loaded with monosodium glutamate, high fructose corn syrup, colors and man-made chemicals. To top it off, then you microwave it in a little plastic container with plastic on top of it. This is combination for illness and disease if eaten often.

If you eat these types of foods, you may lose a bit of weight initially, but inevitably you will gain it back. You will not tone up with this type of food. You need real protein and organic hormone free, artificial free protein shakes, to reshape your body. The chemicals in this food will make you hungrier, which are why when people stop these programs they immediately gain all the weight back, plus more. This is why America is having such a difficult time losing weight and getting healthier. They are overly acidic. Too much acid causes disease and weight gain.

I grew up on a farm in Iowa. I loved the country life. We had fresh meats that we raised, fed, cared for, and knew where it was being processed for us to eat. Now days, our meats may come from overseas, or practiced in large inhumane settings for the benefit of the producer. You don't know what has been injected or fed to these animals that you are now consuming.

On the farm we ate fresh vegetables and fruit all through the year. My mom canned many of our seasonal vegetables and we ate on them all year. Today it is rare you find people living off the land. It is rare you find vegetables or fruit grown without the herbicides, insecticides, or fertilizers. Our food is not the same as it was 30 years ago. Today it is devoid of many minerals, vitamins, nutrients, love, and nurturing as it was then.

Microwaving, artificial sweeteners, high fructose corn syrup, MSG, and antibiotics were not routinely used when I was growing up. Our children are being raised in a different era and an era where the food quality has vanished. The quiet family times are a time of the past since sports and activities have now taken over. People eat on the go. People are now eating fast foods to catch the local football game. We must take time to plan ahead to make our health a priority. We have to schedule health in to our daily calendars.

All truth passes through three stages. First it is ridiculed. Second it is violently opposed. Third it is accepted as self-evident. --Arthur Schopenhauer, German Philosopher

The food industry is in business to make money. Sales are the bottom dollar. They will do whatever they need to market to us, our children. They will add whatever colors, flavor enhancers, addictive substances, and package it in a way to boost sales. This is common business practice. When I was growing up, we had 5 choices of cereal. It was Cheerios, Rice Crispies, Wheaties, Corn Flakes, or Raisin bran. Now days, there are over two hundred cereals. Food, like a drug, increases hunger, and makes people crave and become addicted to certain foods.

The weight loss food industry is estimated to be close to a $150 billion a year market.(Trudeau, 2007) It is important to understand that the multinational corporations involved in the drug industry, food industry, and diet industry are looking at billions of dollars to profit, leaving you and your children to be victims of the SAD (Standard American Diet).

Food companies spend billions of dollars in advertising in virtually every magazine, television network, and radio network. We are inundated with images, words, and phrases to suck us in. Young females fall victim over any other category, as they are the most impressionable.

Mental State of Attitude

Life is all about choices. You have made the choice to start achieving your BETTER BODY. You most likely did not find this book, it found you. You are ready. Make notes in this book. Underline or star the areas you need to take action with. I love the phrase "the teacher appears when the student is ready". Are you ready?

You make choices all day long. The battle of doing what is right, or giving in to what feels or taste good. Most people do know right foods from wrong foods, good thoughts from bad thoughts, and right actions from wrong actions. It's called your conscious. You choose to eat and you make conscious decisions to put unhealthy food into your body. You are aware that certain foods are toxic and are bad for your system, yet you many times choose to continue to eat them. There is no better time than now to stop the vicious cycle.

People, who smoke, know it's bad to smoke. Everyone knows that smoking leads to causes of cancer and is also linked to a series of health and well-being side effects but many still choose to smoke. Even though they know the risks involved and are educated on the health factors on a daily basis, it does not stop people from inhaling. Smoking, alcoholism, drug use; they are all forms of self-abuse.

Food is also another form of abuse that we unleash upon ourselves, and with all addictions, the ripple effects are very far reaching. This touches every part our lives; physical, social, emotional, financial, sexual, spiritual and mental.

Yet with all of the above addictions, you can control them. I will say it again, YOU CAN CONTROL IT. You have a choice over being healthy and you have a choice in becoming healthy. It's the one condition that you CAN control in your life. A person with a debilitating illness sometimes has no choice. However, you have the absolute power over food.

When you are happy, sad, stressed, celebrating, in grief, aroused, elated, food becomes like the alcoholic's chaser. It's part of your everyday life. Why is this? Why has food become such a major part of your makeup? Why do the majority of Americans associate cake, ice-cream, sweets, potato chips, French fries, candy, and chocolate as the GOOD food? Why do you turn to these foods when you are experiencing any type of emotion? How many times have you ever heard anyone saying, "We won the game, let's go eat

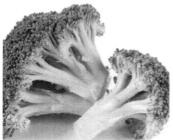

kale and broccoli!!!

You have become accustomed to celebrating with pizza and hamburgers and many times associating happy events with unhealthy foods or beverages. You are conditioned that "comfort" food is the necessary coping mechanism instead of taking a walk, writing in a journal, going to a movie, visiting a loved one, singing, dancing, reading. Why? Because food is quick and it's the quick fix you need at that particular moment.

Overeating and unhealthy eating is like a drug addiction; it's the 'fix' that is never quite fixed. Food literally stimulates the part of your brain that perceives pleasure. The 'high' from the food or cigarettes take over and lasts for five minutes, a half hour, two hours and then the urge happens again and the need to eat and choose something unhealthy takes over yet again. It becomes the bottomless pit that never gets filled. Rest assured, I have answers for you!

The Choice is Yours

You can NEVER make the same mistake TWICE because the second time you make it, it is not a mistake, *it is a choice*.

Once you start living a natural lifestyle, you will start feeling better almost immediately. Your ultimate BETTER BODY transformation is now in the beginning stages. You will soon be able to enjoy the pleasures of life with a body that functions at its peak for years come. Choosing a healthy lifestyle promotes health and happiness in not just your body, but your mind as well.

There are many benefits for those who choose alternative and natural solutions. This includes increased energy, a stronger immune system, faster recovery from illness or injury, and even being more mentally alert.

If you take care of your body, you will never need to resort to quick fixes that are unhealthy, costly or dangerous, to make us better. Staying healthy is the best form of prevention in the process of aging. It's God's plan to see us grow wise and old to the end of our life.

Sometimes, or most of the time maybe, we all get lost in the hustle and bustle of everyday life. Choices and decisions get rushed and the lines between what we need, what we want, and what we're actually doing start to blur. The truth is that although it's great to have all kinds of different goals in life, you have to be careful you're not trying to do too much at once. When is the last time you really thought about your priorities? Not everything can be at the top of the list. Where is your health on that list?

Are you really giving your top priorities the most effort and focus? It seems many people say 'health and losing weight' is a top priority, but then they bog themselves down with so many other things they hardly have time to work on it. Whether you like it or not that means it's at the bottom of the list, not the top.

Why is it that so many of us wait until we experience problems before we try to make changes for our health and well-being? Most of us already have a good basic knowledge about health, yet we tend to push it aside or ignore it.

We eat irregular meals then fill up with all sorts of junk food, we overwork ourselves, we do not get enough rest, we do not keep properly hydrated, we often get little if any exercise, and we continue pushing ourselves even when we are aware that something is wrong until we eventually "burn out." Trust me, I have been there. That is why I am so passionate about getting the message out there.

Our Bodies Need Care and Attention for Our Best Health

1. We need to make sure our brain and the central nervous system is getting all the vital messages to every cell of the body. Chiropractic Adjustments will ensure this.
2. We need to eat the right food types in the correct proportions
3. We need to keep ourselves properly hydrated
4. We need to keep our blood sugars stable
5. We need to keep our hormones well balanced
6. We need to keep our attitude and outlook balanced
7. We need to keep our body alkalized
8. We must keep our body clear of toxins
9. We need to use our whole body - physically and mentally to keep fit
10. We need to get enough sleep
11. We need to schedule in "breaks" and "decompression time" or vacations stay mentally and physically balanced.
12. We need to pay immediate attention to anything that seems wrong

Your total health is far more than just an absence of sickness - it includes every aspect of your life.

There is a big difference between knowing and doing - it only takes a short time to learn something, but it takes a lifetime to put into practice.

We only live once and we only have one "Temple". Respect your "Temple". Care for your body and your "Temple" will reward you with health.

Your health and your life are in YOUR hands. You can make the necessary changes to enhance your health. You can start today. Let's turn the corner together. I am here with you. I will educate you on what it will take to gain a better body and start rebuilding your "Temple".

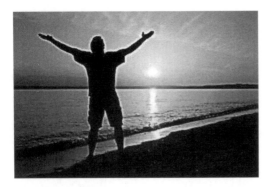

I will give you step by steps on what to do and a system to follow. Live well for your good health! I will take what I have learned over the past 15+ years about health and wellness and give you the basic education so you make smart informed choice to yield your better body!! Let's get started.

Chapter 3

Health is a Cause & Effect Relationship

Before we get into the nuts and bolts of all the solutions, let's look at how optimal health is really a matter of cause and effect. If you do this, then you will get that. It really is that simple and basic.

How do you live, sleep, eat, breathe, and play to live a longer more vibrant health? Adopting a longevity lifestyle, no matter what your age, can help you in your quest for vitality throughout your life. One rule is for certain, what you put into your body will produce the outcome you live. This includes our thoughts, foods, air, medications, words, or activity level.

You must get in the game of health, if you want to win a life of health!!

Every single human cell responds to every single thought you have, every food particle that goes into your body and every activity you partake in. If you truly desire health, there is no better time than now to take action.

Your body is a massive collection of positive and negatively charged cells. Your cells are tiny little microcosms of your body. They know how to breathe, digest, make energy, and respond to certain reactions. They have a life span. Just like you and I, your cells have a typical lifespan. A liver cell lives for 5 months, stomach lining cells live for 2 days, a skin cell lives for 19-34 days, your red blood cells live on average 120 days.(Miller, Cell Lifespan)

"Health is something we do for ourselves, not something that is done to us; a journey rather than a destination; a dynamic, holistic, and purposeful way of living." Dr. Elliot Dacher

What you drink, the choice of foods you put into your body, and your activity levels, and your thought patterns will determine how long you live. Most importantly these factors will determine the quality of life you live.

You can make the choice right now to take back control of your future. The choices you make will not only affect you, but also your family, your family genetic line, your ability to save your money from unplanned diseases.

The CURE is in PREVENTION

What most people don't realize is there is no actual cure for most major diseases! *The cure is in prevention.* The media, the government, teachers, and doctors should be promoting disease prevention. Over 80% of all diseases are preventable.

Imagine if for one decade, only ten years the entire country of America would really focus on lifestyle changes, improving diets, de-stressing, drinking more water, getting more exercise and better sleep. Imagine if all the doctors would teach people about disease prevention. I would estimate you would see a drop in major disease diagnoses by over 50% and trillions of dollars saved.

Instead of running everyone through thousands of tests and putting people on trillions of dollars of medications, we would educate people on health. What would our world be like in one decade's time if we would teach health to our kids, we would feed our kids healthy foods, we would promote wellness care, rather than sickness care. What if the government would actually pay for vitamins, herbs, minerals, healthy foods, exercise programs, acupuncture, detoxing, massages, and natural health methods? What would happen? How would our world change?

I can only keep on praying for that day to come. Until then, let me guide you on the steps necessary to take back your future longevity.

How Quickly Can You Achieve Your BETTER BODY?

Human nature is immediate gratification. We all want to feel good today. We want the weight to fall off now. We want the pain to go away yesterday. We are looking for quick fixes. Our society has programmed us to fast food, instant meals, microwave, fast speed internet; drive through, pick up, drop off, instant mail, constant contact, immediate results, and electronics have only made it worse. Nothing is worse than waiting more than 10 seconds for a page to open up on a computer browser. If our computers are too slow, people get antsy.

> *Statistics show that for every hour you exercise, you add two hours to your life.*

As your Holistic Health coach, I am here to break the news to you. Health does not work that way. Weight loss does not work that way. It may take some time. But rest assured, with consistency, baby steps, and a positive attitude you will yield remarkable results with your new better body.

The Following Will Contribute to How Quickly You See Results With Your BETTER BODY:

1. What is your age?
2. What are your stress levels?
3. How many medical or health conditions do you have?
4. Whether you like your job or not?
5. Is your occupation physically demanding?
6. Are you properly hydrated?

7. Are you on any medications?
8. How is your diet, what is the quality of your food you consume?
9. What type of people do you hang around (healthy or unhealthy…..fit or fat…..negative or positive)?
10. Do you take good nutritional supplements, these help you rebuild the inside of your body?
11. Do you exercise?
12. Do you eat many sugars, white starchy products, or carbohydrates?
13. Do you eat sweets, candy, or pop?
14. Do you stretch regularly?
15. How are your bowel habits?
16. Do you eat at regular hours?
17. How well do you sleep?
18. Do you smoke?
19. Do you do drugs?
20. Are you a happy person or a negative person?
21. If female, where are you at with your monthly cycle or are you going through menopause?
22. Do you consume alcohol?
23. Do you consume caffeine?
24. If in a relationship, is it a healthy supportive one?
25. Where do you live? Is it full of poor air quality and do you have to deal with heavy traffic?
26. How often do you find time for YOU time, or to relax?
27. How busy is your lifestyle?
28. Are you toxic? Have you ever done a detox program?
29. Have you been on numerous antibiotics?
30. Any illnesses, infections, or bad injuries?
31. Do you sit in front of computers or electronics all day?
32. *And the most important question*…. How bad do you want to improve? Are you willing to make some changes?

So as you can see, health truly is a cause and effect relationship. This process will take some time. So be patient. The more factors you have against you, the longer it may take to bring you back to health. You know your health is one of your most prized possessions. As without it, you can't enjoy your family, your children, your home, your cars, your vacations, and all the other "things". The effort you put into your mental and physical health is equivalent to what you will get out of it. Now is your chance. Take the step towards a better body, a better you, and a better life. If you put steps in action, you will yield the outcome you desire. Your "Temple" will be strong and beautiful.

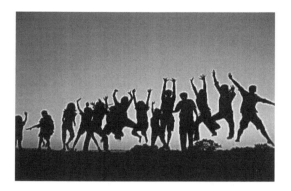

Chapter 4

The Role of Proper Nutrition

TO EAT or NOT TO EAT,

That is the Question

"For too long nutrition has been denied its proper role in American medicine. Billions are spent on disease each year, but very little is spent on nutrition, which is often the key for preventing disease. Few doctors have the time or inclination to teach those aspects of diet which are essential to their patient's well-being." Moin Ansari, Ph. D., Nutritionist.

"Whatever you eat or drink or whatever you do, you must do all for the glory of God" 1 Corinthians 10:31

Let's think of two scenarios for a moment. You have two ladies buying groceries for their families in the same market. They both love their families. They both are nice ladies who mean well for their families. They both grew up in the same town, and do many of the same activities. We will call them Mary and Sue.

Mary passes by the fresh produce, buys boxed meals, buys pop tarts, sugary colored juices, canned fruit, a few cans of green beans, boxes of cereal, hot dogs, nuggets, chips, three 12 packs of soda, white wonder bread, coffee, ice cream, lunchables, pre-packed cold cuts, pre-made mashed potatoes, jars of gravy, canned soups, regular milk, sugar free jello, sugar free whipped cream, and she can't forget the loads of air fresheners, fragranced laundry soap, and bottles of disinfectants. Her family doesn't feel the best most times. Her kids are on medication for ADD/ ADHD. She is on anti-depressants and laxatives from being constipated. Her husband is overweight, has diabetes and high blood pressure. He is on 4 different medications. She and her husband both need sleeping pills each night.

Now Sue has been an avid health conscious woman. She reads and becomes educated on what to feed her family and how certain foods are contributing to her family feeling healthy and alive. She spends most of her time on the perimeters of the market, where all the "fresh" and perishable foods are located. She buys every color of fresh fruit, and it must be organic. She buys a variety of colors of fresh vegetables. As vegetables are a main staple in her families diet. She buys organic preservative free salad dressing, stops by the deli for fresh cut organic nitrate free turkey or chicken. She rarely buys red meat. She buys fresh organic chicken. She also buys fresh fish. She buys whole grain pastas. She buys lots of variety of nuts and seeds for her family to snack on. She buys fresh organic eggs, organic milk, almond milk, and organic Greek yogurts. She also buys fresh made whole grain bread from the bakery. No fake potatoes for Sue, she buys fresh potatoes and boils them and freshly mashes. She uses organic butter and olive oil to cook with. She buys bottled spring water. She buys fragrance free laundry soap, organic and minimally colored foods. She looks for things with short ingredient lists. She buys baking soda and vinegar for her cleaning solutions. She buys lots of fresh lemons for water and also cleaning solutions. She also buys dark chocolate for her families treats.

To continue with Sue, she buys fresh popcorn that she uses her stir crazy popcorn popper and olive oil to cook with. No bagged popcorn for Sue, she understands all the chemicals in the bagged popcorn. She buys Fresh tomatoes, basil, and garlic and makes her own spaghetti sauce. She also buys steel cut oats. She uses stevia as her family's sweetener instead of sugar. Raisins are also on her list. Finally, she buys fresh blocks of minimally processed cheese that she freshly grates. Additionally, she grows her own garden, herbs, and shops the local farmers market each week. Her family feels great! They sleep great too. No medication for anyone in this family and it has been years since anyone needed to go to the doctor's office for any health concerns.

As you can see this is the division of America's philosophical living choices. Sue is educated on how food affects her family and Mary is not. Both are great women, but Sue's family will feel better; have more money in the bank from less medication and doctor's visits. They both spend about the same, just focused completely different. My hope is you become a shopper more like Sue.

Step one in getting your BETTER BODY is healthy eating. What is "Nutrition"? It is the building blocks for your entire health and physical makeup. What you eat determines the quantity and quality of your life. Food is fuel for your body. Many researchers show strong evidence that food and nutrition is a high indicator for immune system strength, emotional well-being, disease resistance, and overall longevity.

Ironically, look where America's values are when it comes to purchases in the grocery stores. According to Information Resources Inc.:

Top 10 Items Purchased at Grocery Stores

1. Carbonated/Sugary Beverages
2. Milk
3. Fresh Breads & Rolls
4. Beer/Ale/ Hard Cider
5. Salty Snacks
6. Natural Cheese
7. Frozen Dinners/Entrees
8. Cold Cereal

9.   Wine
10.   Cigarettes

Some telling things that jump out on this list are the things that are missing, such as vegetables, fruits, healthy fats and meats & beans. The other important thing that jumps out is how much of this list is highly processed 'foods', including sodas, snacks and frozen dinners. Our country needs education on HEALTH!!! At this rate how much longer can the human race last??? We are slowly killing ourselves from the foods we are eating. The sad thing is sometimes there are no healthy options even available, such as your children or grandchildren's school lunches.

Let me warn you, sadly it may cost less to eat unhealthy rather than healthy. What is wrong with this picture? Many times to buy organic food options it may cost more. Here is what I say to that, either you pay a little extra now or you will pay later. By spending the extra money on healthy foods, high quality foods, and nutrients it is like insurance for your future health. Additionally, you will feel better, have more energy and have an increase in the quality of your life.

Optimum Diet

Your optimum diet should be abundant in FRESH (raw) fruits and vegetables. Many experts agree the Mediterranean type diet is one of the best consisting of: fish, veggies, fruits, lentils, legumes, seeds, nuts, whole grains, complex carbohydrates, good fats, minimal red meats, do minimal sugars and starchy pastas every other day to reduce overexposure to high insulin levels.

Fresh raw organic, unprocessed fruits and vegetables are always the best source of nutrients. They are packed full of vitamins, minerals, enzymes, color, flavor, fiber, and hydration. They are God's living foods to keep the human race alive. We need more of them.

Water:

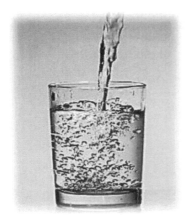

- Drink ½ your body weight in ounces per day.
- A minimum would be 6-8 glasses (not cups) per day.
- Have it be spring water or filtered water.

Vegetables:

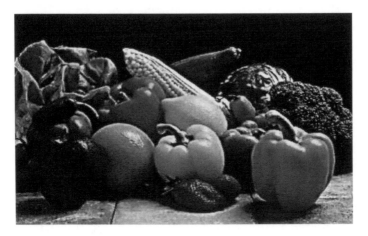

- Raw is best.
- Fresh, organic is best.
- Eat a variety of colors. (Carrots, peas, asparagus, tomatoes, corn, cucumbers, beets, etc.)
- Have one large spinach or fresh greens salad per day with a variety of veggies
- Have 4-6 additional ½-1 cup servings of other veggies. Steaming or grilled is OK. Use olive oil as a topping.

Fruit:

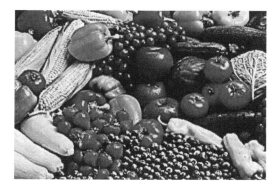

- Raw is best.
- Fresh, Organic is best.
- Eat a variety of colors. (Apples, blueberries, strawberries, oranges, pineapple, plums, etc.)
- Have fruit at least every other day and eat your fruit earlier in the day for weight management. Fruit later in the day will spike your blood sugar and leave you prone to weight gain.

Dairy:

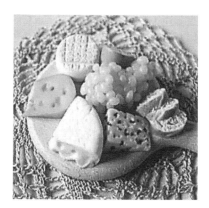

- Use sparingly.
- Use organic milk, eggs, cheese, yogurt if having dairy.
- Have 2-3 servings per day.

Starches:

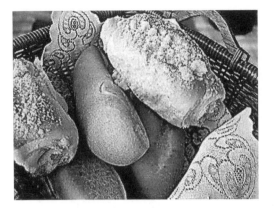

- Use whole grains. Eliminate as much white flour and white sugar products as possible.
- Use raw and/or organic as much as possible.
- Avoid white sugar or floury products (pretzels, pastries, buns, crackers, chips, cookies, doughnuts)
- Avoid high fructose corn syrup products.
- Oatmeal, rye, whole wheat, quinoa products are good.
- I prefer to keep starches to a minimum. We can get our carbohydrates from fruits and vegetables.
- Get at least 30-40 grams of fiber in per day (look at the food labels)

Meats/ Proteins:

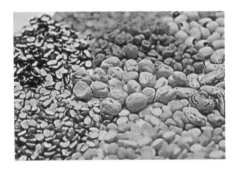

- Use sparingly
- Use organic, non-hormone, non-antibiotic meats
- Use lean (90-93%) if using red meats.
- Choose chicken, turkey, fish for daily serving.

- Consume minimal red meats.
- 3-4 ounces is a serving.
- Use nuts, seeds, lentils, legumes, beans often as protein source (non-meat sources).

Fats:

- Use extra-virgin olive oil daily
- Use 2-3 table spoons olive oil daily.
- Use 1-2 tablespoons of ground organic flax seed daily. (coffee bean grinder works great)
- Use butters sparingly, no margarine.
- Snack on almonds, peanuts, avocados, seeds as a source of "good fats"
- Use coconut oil 3-4 times per week to cook with.
- Peanut butter or almond butter is a great snack on whole grain rice cakes.

Sweets/ Others:

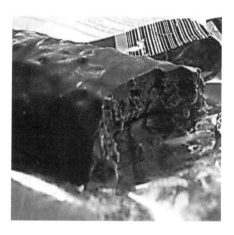

- Use minimally (weekly, not daily).
- Consume fruit to satisfy your sweet tooth.
- Use stevia as your sweetener.
- Use honey or Agave nectar as sweeteners.
- Dark chocolate 70% or higher
- Granola mixes are better than candy

Other Areas of Concern with Foods

Use your food as fuel. Think of everything you put into your mouth. *Is it contributing to your health or stealing your health?* Most people inherently know the answer. Do not eat in front of TV. Stop eating before 7 pm. Do not drink liquids with your meals. Avoid Fast Foods. Avoid Fried foods. Avoid all sodas. Use green teas or pure water for liquids. Don't use food for emotional comfort.

Two Main Basic Diet Categories:

Macro and Micro Diets

Macro Diets: Carbohydrates, Fats, Proteins

Low glycemic index (converts to blood sugar slowly= digestive enzymes have time to break it down how nature intended). Examples: nuts, beans, legumes, fruits, blueberries, apricots, whole grains.

High glycemic index (processed foods, cereals, breads) = rapid rise in blood sugar (due to processing breaking it down for us) = pancreas releases insulin = clears sugar from the blood= weight gain, obesity, diabetes (if you have a genetic history of this you are extremely high risk).

Glycemic Index

The glycemic index was formulated in 1981 in Canada. The reason for inventing the glycemic index was to determine the impact that carbs have on blood sugar levels. It was found to have significant effect on human's health especially for diabetics.

The Glycemic Index (GI) is a ranking of carbohydrates on a scale from 0 to 100 according to the extent to which they raise blood sugar levels after eating. Low GI diets have been shown to improve both glucose and lipid levels in people with diabetes (type 1 and type 2).

Low Glycemic Index Foods

- Low fat meats- beef, skinless chicken, pork, lamb
- Seafood – mussels, oysters, lobsters
- Fish
- Fresh fruits – orange, grapefruits, apples, berries, cherries, grapes, apricots, melon, watermelon, kiwi, pineapples, papaya, cantaloupe, pear
- Vegetables – broccoli, raw carrots, cauliflower, cabbages, tomatoes, artichokes, bean sprouts, soybeans, peas, radishes, asparagus, onion, radishes, olives

- Breads and Cereals – wheat, rye, whole grains, multi-grain, rice bran oats
- Starch – couscous, brown rice, lentils, whole-wheat pastas
- Dairy – low-fat milk, low-fat/fat-free cheese, low-fat/sugar-free yogurt, tofu, low-fat cottage cheese, egg whites
- Beverages – water, diet colas, sugar-free drinks, tea, coffee, both without sugar and milk/cream

High Glycemic Index Foods

- Fried chicken with skin
- Duck
- Bacon, Hotdogs, Hamburgers
- Fatty meats
- Liver, Liverwurst
- Conserved fish/seafood in oil
- Fruits – canned fruits, bananas, dates, coconut, mangoes, and sweetened fruit juices, dried fruits, raisins, marmalade
- Vegetables – cooked carrots, avocado, beets, olives in oil, corn, potatoes, parsnips, sweet pickles
- Cereals and bread- white bread, bagels, chips, biscuits, croissants, cookies, cakes, pastries, muffins, waffles, popcorn
- Starch – white pasta, baked or fried beans, white or fried rice, ramen noodles, pretzels, soups unless vegetable broth
- Dairy – cheese high in fat, cream cheese, sorbet, ice cream, frozen yogurt
- Beverages – any sweetened drinks, alcoholic drinks

Fats

It is an essential nutrient and each gram contains 9 calories. Fats should be 30% of your diet. It is about the kind of fat you consume that you should be concerned with, fat is not bad, we need healthy fats to be healthy.

Saturated fats: hard in room temp. Butter, cheese, dairy, (Americans diet) Keep to less than 5% of your diet.

Poly: nuts and seeds. Liquid at room temperature. Chemically unstable. Produces inflammation. Corn, safflower. Keep to around 5% of your diet.

Mono: olive (liquid room temp, but as the temp drops it turns thicker). Mono unsaturated fats: best type. Grape seed oil. 20%

Strictly Avoid: margarine, any whipped unnatural spreads. Trans fat, hydrogenated oils. Chips, pastries, crackers, cookies. Look at labels.

Fat typically has a very satisfying component to your taste buds. The less fat, you lose the desirable taste. The right type of fat is healthy for you and needed for your cell membranes, skin, hormones, and brain function. Keep in mind, the right healthy fats, not the fast fried food fats.

Omega fatty acids: fish, flaxseed protects from cancer, inflammation, and certain diseases.

Do not eat deep fried foods; they are oxidized and completely unhealthy for you. These fats are not changed very often.

Good Fats: Avocado, pistachios, nuts, seeds, natural peanut butters, walnuts, most seeds, olive oils.

Chocolate: fat in the cocoa butter is handled like olive oil. High quality dark chocolates are best. Fat is not evil in and of itself. If you get too low in fat when cooking, you will not have a desirable meal.

Proteins

The bodies needs for protein is much smaller than we think. Growing children, nursing mothers, pregnant mothers, injury recovery, and athletes all need the most protein.

Consuming protein will put a great work load on your digestion system. Many times I recommend extra digestive enzymes to help break down your protein intake. Most people are deficient in adequate digestive enzymes due to stress, medications, age, and poor nutrition. The liver and kidneys have to work hard to process proteins.

I recommend 50-100 grams per day as a target for people. Another way to look at it is half your body weight in grams per day of protein. If you are an athlete or working out hard, I recommend more.

Eat more vegetable proteins or fish, nuts, beans as a good source of protein. If you use chicken or beef get hormone free or antibiotic free.

Minimize cured meats (nitrates / nitrates= carcinogen) such as bacon, hot dogs, nuggets. These are highly processed and contain additional colors, preservatives, chemicals, and loaded with salts. There has been research linking cured meats with attention problems in children, many times due to the MSG.

Diary: Be cautious of cow's milk (extremely high allergen) until 2 years old. Use soy or alternate. Toddlers DO NOT need cow's milk all throughout the day. Keep to a minimum. Use almond milk, water, low sugar juices.

Micro Nutrient Diet: vitamins, minerals, and plant sources

If we eat the optimum diet we should be able to get our vitamins, however we typically do not get the optimum diet.

We should not skip real foods if we take supplements, because nothing can replace the nutrients we receive from real foods.

Although only needed in small amounts, vitamins are important contributors to the body's daily functions and are essential to its growth and repair. They are considered essential because the body does not produce vitamins naturally, and they must be obtained from food. Most discoveries about the human need for essential vitamins were made as a direct result of their deficiency.

> *If you are interested in healthy eating, avoid shopping in the center aisles and end caps of the grocery store. The healthy choices are on the perimeter of the store.*

Because of high bioavailability it is best to obtain vitamins from food. Whole foods contain vitamins and other trace minerals that are more easily digested and absorbed into the bloodstream.

Vitamins

	Possible Benefits	Best Sources
VITAMIN A Beta-Carotene	Beta-carotene is converted to vitamin A, which helps cells develop, advances bone and tooth growth, and boosts the body's immune system. You also need vitamin A to help you see at night.	You're well on your way to getting enough if you regularly eat dairy products and eggs. Leafy green vegetables, carrots, broccoli, cantaloupe, peaches, and squash are also great sources.
VITAMIN B-6	B-6 helps the body process proteins, fats, and carbohydrates. Works with other vitamins and minerals to supply energy to the muscles. Aids in the production of blood cells. Important for a healthy immune system.	Chicken, fish, pork, liver, eggs, spinach, potatoes, bananas, whole wheat bread, and peanut butter – the list is so long and varied that most people don't have to worry about getting enough.
VITAMIN B-12	B-12 helps the body use fats and carbohydrates. Important in cell development, especially blood cells. Also helps the nervous system work properly.	Meats, chicken, fish, and dairy products are great sources.
VITAMIN C	Vitamin C is needed to produce collagen, which makes up connective tissue. Acts as an antioxidant, protecting cells from natural destruction that occurs with aging. Not proven to prevent colds, but studies have found that big doses – around 2,000 mg a day- can make cold symptoms milder.	If you eat fruits and vegetables every day – especially citrus fruits, broccoli, leafy greens, red and green peppers – you're probably getting enough.
VITAMIN D	Vitamin D regulates the formation and repair of bone and cartilage. It also controls the amount of calcium and phosphorus you absorb from foods.	If you drink milk regularly, you're getting plenty. Your body also forms vitamin D when exposed to the sun. Older men and women should consider daily supplements to protect their bones.
VITAMIN E	Vitamin E appears highly effective in preventing heart disease. It is an anti-oxidant, protecting cells from natural destruction that occurs with aging. Helps prevent blood clots. Needed for red blood cell production.	Nuts, meats, leafy green vegetables and vegetable oil. Most Americans get enough to meet the R.D.A. To protect the heart, a 400 IU daily supplement is best.
FOLIC ACID	Low folic acid levels increase your risk of dying from coronary heart disease. Also regulates embryo and fetal development: Low levels increase a woman's chance of having a baby with neurological defects. Needed for red blood production.	If you eat lots of leafy greens, peas, beans, citrus fruits, or whole grain breads, you are probably getting enough. Women planning on pregnancy should make sue to eat plenty of these foods or take a supplement to prevent birth defects.
NIACIN	Niacin aids in processing fat and producing sugar. It helps tissues get rid of waste materials. It also lowers cholesterol levels in the blood, reducing the risk of heart disease.	Plentiful in meats, niacin is also formed in the body form proteins in eggs and milk.

Minerals

The body needs these!! You will want to take these to achieve a better body and start healing your Temple.

It can be overwhelming if going to a health food store and seeing all the different vitamins and minerals.

Mineral	Best Sources	Functions
CALCIUM	Dairy products, spinach, kale, okra, collards, and white beans.	Strong bones, teeth, muscle tissue; regulated heartbeat, muscle action, and nerve function; blood clotting.
CHROMIUM	Brewer's yeast, lean meats, cheeses, pork kidney, whole-grain breads and cereals, molasses, spices, and some bran cereals	Glucose metabolism (energy); increases effectiveness of insulin to regulate blood sugar levels
COPPER	Oysters and other shellfish, whole grains, beans, nuts, potatoes, and organ meats, dark leafy greens.	Formation of red blood cells; bone growth and health; works with vitamin C to form elastin.
IODINE	Seafood, iodized salt	Component of hormone thyroxin, which controls metabolism.
IRON	Dried beans, dried fruits, eggs, liver, lean red meat, oysters, salmon, tuna, whole grains	Hemoglobin formation; improves blood quality; increases resistance to stress and disease.
MAGNESIUM	Nuts, green vegetables, whole grains	Acid/alkaline balance; important in metabolism of carbs, minerals, and sugar(glucose)
MANGANESE	Nuts, whole grains, vegetables and fruits.	Enzyme activation; carbohydrate and fat production; sex hormone production; skeletal development
MOLYBDENUM	Legumes, grain products and nuts.	Functions as a cofactor for a limited number of enzymes in humans.
PHOSPHORUS	Fish, meat, poultry, eggs and grains.	Bone development; important in protein, fat and carb utilization.
POTASSIUM	Lean meat, vegetables and fruits.	Fluid balance; controls activity of heart muscle, nervous system and kidneys.
SELENIUM	Seafood, organ meats, lean meats and grains.	Protects body tissues against oxidative damage from radiation pollution, and normal metabolic processing
ZINC	Lean meats, liver, eggs, seafood and whole grains.	Involved in digestion and metabolism; development of reproductive system.

Fiber

Proper amounts of fiber in your diet will help your body to move indigestible foods and bulk up your stool. Low fiber is hard for bowel elimination.

Dietary fibers are found naturally in the plants that we eat. They are parts of plant that do not break down in our stomachs, and instead pass through our system undigested. All dietary fibers are either soluble or insoluble. Both types of fiber are equally important for health, digestion, and preventing conditions such as heart disease, diabetes, obesity, diverticulitis, and constipation.

There are two kinds of fiber soluble and insoluble.

Soluble fibers: attract water and form a gel, which slows down digestion. Soluble fiber delays the emptying of your stomach and makes you feel full, which helps control weight. Slower stomach emptying may also affect blood sugar levels and have a beneficial effect on insulin sensitivity, which may help control diabetes. Soluble fibers can also help lower LDL ("bad") blood cholesterol by interfering with the absorption of dietary cholesterol.

    Sources of soluble fiber: oatmeal, oat cereal, lentils, apples, oranges, pears, oat bran, strawberries, nuts, flaxseeds, beans, dried peas, blueberries, psyllium, cucumbers, celery, and carrots.

Insoluble fibers: are considered gut-healthy fiber because they have a laxative effect and add bulk to the diet, helping prevent constipation. These fibers do not dissolve in water, so they pass through the gastrointestinal tract relatively intact, and speed up the passage of food and waste through your gut. Insoluble fibers are mainly found in whole grains and vegetables.

    Sources of insoluble fiber: whole wheat, whole grains, wheat bran, corn bran, seeds, nuts, barley, couscous, brown rice, bulgur, zucchini, celery, broccoli, cabbage, onions, tomatoes, carrots, cucumbers, green beans, dark leafy vegetables, raisins, grapes, fruit, and root vegetable skins.

Fiber slows down conversion of blood sugars. Your goal of fiber intake should be **40 grams per day**.

Phytochemicals

Chances are you've eaten phytochemicals. Don't be scared -- they're not toxic agents produced by some huge chemical company, as the name might suggest. Phytochemicals are natural compounds found in the fruits and vegetables we eat (or should eat) every day.

Phytochemicals help give an orange its orange color and make a strawberry red. More importantly, they may protect us from some of the most deadly diseases that threaten us -- diseases such as cancer and heart disease.

The term "phytochemicals" refers to a wide variety of compounds produced by plants. They are found in fruits, vegetables, beans, grains, and other plants. Scientists have identified thousands of phytochemicals, although only a small fraction have been studied closely. Some of the more commonly known phytochemicals include beta carotene, ascorbic acid (vitamin C), folic acid, and vitamin E.

Proper nutrition is one of the key components to creating a more shapely body. The foods you put in your body will account for up to 80% of you physique.

Phytochemicals originated to help plants survive in an often hostile environment. When the Earth was young, there was very little free oxygen in the atmosphere. Plants, which take in carbon dioxide and release oxygen, eventually increased the oxygen composition. But by doing so, they polluted their own environment. To protect themselves from the highly reactive oxygen, plants developed antioxidant compounds, including phytochemicals. Today, thanks to these antioxidants, plants can survive -- and thrive -- in our oxygen-rich environment. Phytochemicals also protect plants against bacteria, fungi, viruses and cell damage. The same phytochemicals that protect plants also help the humans who eat them.

There are hundreds -- maybe even thousands -- of different phytochemicals contained in fruits and vegetables.

Food	Phytochemicals	Benefits
Apples	Flavonoids	Protect against cancer, lower cholesterol
Beans	Flavonoids (saponins)	Protect against cancer, lower cholesterol
Berries	Ellagic acid	Prevent abnormal cellular changes that can lead to cancer
Broccoli	Indoles, isothiocyanates	Protect against cancer, heart disease and stroke
Carrots	Beta-carotene	Antioxidant
Citrus fruits	Flavonoids (limonene)	Antioxidant, inhibit tumor formation, decrease inflammation
Flaxseed	Isoflavones	Protect against cancer, lower cholesterol
Garlic	Allium (allyl sulfides)	Protect against certain cancers and heart disease, boost the immune system
Grains	Isoflavones	Protect against cancer, lower cholesterol
Red grapes (and wine)	Flavonoids (quercetin)	Protect against cancer and heart disease
Onions	Allium (allyl sulfides)	Protect against certain cancers and heart disease, boost the immune system
Sweet potatoes	Beta-carotene	Antioxidant
Soy (soybeans)	Isoflavones	Protect against cancer and heart disease, strengthen bones
Tea	Flavonoids (quercetin)	Protect against cancer and heart disease
Tomatoes	Flavonoids	Protect against cancer, fight infection

Phytochemicals protects us from cancers and environmental toxins.

These God given healing properties in our foods are found in the reds, purples, dark green foods, broccoli, deep yellows, and soy.

VARY Your Fruits and Vegetables

Teas: Tannins: Green teas: strong preventative for cancer, heart disease, 4 cups per day is desirable.

Red wine: heart protective: red pigments, not alcohol

Chocolate: dark: antioxidant

Mushrooms: Immune enhancement, evidence is strong, not super market, shitake, mitake & Asian mushrooms.

Water: Is the most important nutrient we need!! Use bottled water or get a home purifier.

Optimum (high quality) fuel/ nutrition = Optimum health

Body chemistry is the sum of all the metabolic functions plus what we put into the body (foods, liquids, toxins, etc.)

Body Chemistry is Dependent Upon

1. Our environment: food, drinks, air, state of mind, stress level.

2. Body function: reactions to our environment, healing ability, assimilation, digestion, circulation, hormones, blood sugar stability, detoxification ability, sleep.

Food: has an Acid or Alkaline Effect on the Body and is Based on Mineral / Nutrient profile

1. Alkaline foods are higher in K, Na, Mg, Ca (fruits and veggies)
2. Acid foods are higher in S, P, fats, carbs (fats, starches, proteins)
3. Blood pH must be kept between 7.35-7.45
4. The body has several buffering mechanisms to maintain balance. When we don't take in enough alkaline forming nutrients, the body starts to break down to release necessary nutrients to buffer acids. When this happens over time, we develop symptoms.
5. Depletion of our alkaline/ buffering reserves causes the body to liberate alkaline nutrients from tissues/ bones which causes breakdown and illnesses.
6. 70% food should be alkaline (3/4 of your plate veggies/fruit) and only 30% should be acidic (1/4 of your plate meat, starch, or fats).

Are you heading for an acidic body? Take charge before it's too late!! We will be talking about this in a later chapter. Be sure to find out about the acid-alkaline balance and how it contributes to health and longevity.

Do We Need Supplements?

In many instances, yes we do need supplements, due to our poor food quality and poor food choices. Also due to our intense stress loads and poor health conditions. Many of the medications people are taking, depletes your body of nutrients. Our body is constantly battling the environment and physical demands. Supplements help to balance and support. They can also be viewed as a way to REBUILD and REPAIR the body.

Make sure they are pharmaceutical grade, high quality, organic, strict regulations to follow, scientific research to back it up.

Food: Why We Need It?

We need food for energy, repair and for fuel. To grow we need fuel. To lose weight we need the right fuel. We will die without food. We will get diseases and conditions if we do not get the right foods. If we have an extremely healthy balanced diet free of sugar, flour, and preservatives you will have minimal pain or health conditions.

Chew at least 30 times before swallowing. Do not drink liquids with meals as this dilutes your digestive enzymes.

What Types of Food are Best?

Do not eat : white sugar products, white flour products, high fructose corn syrup, dyes, MSG, "diet" foods or beverages with sucralose or aspartame (excitatory/ neurotoxin), limit dairy, limit hormone and antibiotic filled meat products, high sodium foods, preservatives, boxed foods, and processed foods.

Do eat: fresh or raw fruits, vegetables, nuts, seeds, organic eggs, organic hormone free lean meats, legumes, lentils, beans, granolas, oatmeal, rye, brown rice, homemade foods, low fats, olive oils, fresh and organic foods, olives, olive oils.

Healing Foods or "Super Foods"

Super Foods includes broccoli, garlic, blueberries, oatmeal, tomatoes, papaya, asparagus, spinach, apples, walnuts, white fish, fresh fruits, fresh veggies, nuts, lentils, beans.

How Much Food Do You Need?

Men: 2000-2300 calories per day approx. (depends on activity level)

Women: 1700-2100 calories per day approx. (depends on activity)

Emotional Eating

The first step in this area is awareness!! Realize when you are actually hungry versus emotionally filling a void. Have your "anchor" that you use when you are emotional. Reach for what keeps you focused and grounded. Perhaps a glass of water, going for a walk, giving yourself a "timeout" in your quiet spot, your bag of carrots or a piece of gum. Many extra calories add up to lots of extra pounds from boredom or anxiety to achieve your BETTER BODY, **You do have control. This takes discipline. You are a disciplined person.**

Save your eating for meal time. Be realistic, it is all about balance. Cultural eating can be challenging. As with certain cultures it is centered on eating and celebrating with delicious high calorie meals. Perhaps try to eat ahead of time on lower calorie foods before going to the celebration. Also perhaps you could bring a dish with fresh vegetables or a delicious homemade salad.

Water as a Nutrient

Functions of water in the body: transports nutrients, cellular activity, healthy mucous membranes, lubricates joints, regulates body temperature, and removes toxins, cell communication, electrical impulses, and immune system fuel.

You need pure water. Not flavored. Drink half your body in ounces (200 pounds = 100 oz.) Your urine should be clear and you should go every few hours.

We are typically not told that many of our lifestyle and dietary habits induce DEHYDRATION (caffeine, alcohol, processed foods, smoking, exercise, low humidity, sweating.)

DEHYDRATION HAS MANY HEALTH CONSEQUENCES!!!!

Healthy eating starts with the right attitude. First, let's remember that the purpose of food is to fuel and nourish the body. It is also for our enjoyment and pleasure. However, it is not meant to take center stage in our lives, consuming much of our thoughts and emotional energy. The goal is overall healthful eating, without having to obsess over every bite. It requires some planning and a little effort, but is not a complicated, exhausting process. With the right attitude, healthful eating becomes a way of life, not another diet to go on and off.

One of the important things you can do for your overall health is to eat a healthy diet. Your diet affects your weight and increases your risks of health diseases. Deciding a healthy diet is easier to say than to do because it is tempting to eat less healthy foods. No one diet works for everyone, since we are all unique individuals we have to find the combination that works best.

Healthy eating means establishing good habits. First, examine your eating patterns. Do you tend to eat erratically, often skipping meals? If so, you've learned that this only leads to extreme hunger and uncontrolled eating at the end of the day. The first good habit to set is eating three balanced meals a day, with healthy snacks in between as needed. This keeps the body supplied with a steady source of fuel. In addition to regular eating, where and how we eat are equally important. Do you frequently find yourself wolfing down your dinner in the car, munching in front of the TV, or grabbing snacks as you stand at the refrigerator door? We need to incorporate calmer eating practices, such as sitting at the table without distractions, so we can enjoy our food.

Healthy eating means variety and moderation. This advice may sound boring, but the key to good health is eating something from all food groups, in moderation. Carbohydrates, proteins and fats ALL play important roles in maintaining a healthy body. Eating a variety of types of foods also ensures that we're supplying our bodies with all the necessary vitamins and minerals. Any diet plans that require eliminating lists of foods or whole groups are going to be lacking in certain nutrients, and are also not realistic in the long run.

Healthy eating requires listening to your body. This means to retrain our bodies to eat when we are hungry, and stop when we are comfortably full– neither denying ourselves of food nor overstuffing.

Healthy eating incorporates healthy choices. Without a doubt, fruits and vegetables are rich in phytochemicals which help fight heart disease, cancer and premature aging. They are also power-packed with nutrients, yet relatively low in calories. A diet rich in fruits, vegetables, beans and whole grains is both nutritious and satisfying.

Healthy eating means putting food in its place. Isn't it amazing that food, which is not even alive, can wield so much power in our lives? We comfort, medicate, celebrate, entertain, procrastinate and companion ourselves with food. Instead, we need to find healthy alternatives to meet our emotional needs, manage stress, and enrich our lives.

Healthy eating results in good health. With a goal of eating well for a healthy body, we are freed from the restrictive mindset that dieting fosters. Weight will fall at what is healthiest for our own individual body types. With proper nourishment and adequate fuel, we have more energy, think more clearly and function more efficiently.

With healthy eating, we are free to experience the joys and blessings of life.

> *"Your body is a temple of the HOLY SPIRIT, who is in you, whom you have received from God. You are not your own; you were bought at a price therefore honor God with your bodies." 1 Corinthians 6:19-20*

Chapter 5

Balanced Blood Sugars, Avoiding Sugar

The second step moving you towards your BETTER BODY is stabilizing your blood sugars and learning about how sugar affects your health and weight.

For most of us, sugar is a symbol of love and nurturance, because as infants, our first food is lactose, or milk sugar. Overconsumption and daily use of sugar is the first compulsive habit for most everyone. Simple sugar, or glucose, is what our body, our cells, and our brain use as fuel for energy. Excess sugar is stored as fat for use during periods of low-calorie intake or starvation.

Problems with sweets come from the frequency we eat them and the quantity we consume. The type of sugar we eat is also a contributing factor.

Sugar and sweeteners have become so integrated into our food manufacturing and restaurant industries that it is almost impossible to find prepackaged products that are unsweetened. Both refined, high-calorie, non-nutrient sucrose and corn syrup derivatives, mainly as high-fructose corn syrup.

Many nutritional authorities feel that the high use of sugar in our diet is a significant underlying cause of disease. Too much sweetener in any form can have a negative effect on our health; this includes not only refined sugar, but also corn syrup, honey, fruit juices, and treats such as sodas, cakes and candies. Because sugary foods satisfy our hunger, they often replace more nutritious foods and weaken our tissue's health and disease fighting abilities.

This is the one area of my practice where I focus a lot of time educating people. You must understand sugar can be a contributing factor to causing disease. It can cause all diseases to last longer and never have a fighting chance for recovery. Sugar weakens our immune function. Sugar causes problems with biochemistry if consumed too often. I tell people keep it to 30-50 grams per day or less. Have it come from natural fruit sources. And whatever you do don't switch to artificial chemically altered sugar, in the pink, blue, or yellow packets. Use Stevia or Xylitol as natural sweeteners. You may use honey or agave nectar as well. Organic cane sugar may be used in moderation.

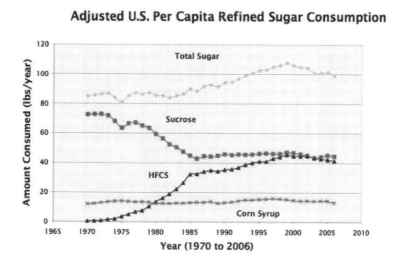

Adjusted U.S. Per Capita Refined Sugar Consumption

Sugar on Your Brain and Body

We consume an enormous amount of sugar, whether consciously or not, but it's a largely misunderstood substance. There are different kinds and different ways your body processes them all. Some consider it poison and others believe it's the sweetest thing on earth. Here's a look at the different forms of sugar, the various ways they affect you, and how they play a role in healthy—and unhealthy—diets.

Not Simply Sugar

Glucose is a simple sugar that your body likes. Your cells use it as a primary source of energy, so when you consume glucose, it's actually helpful. When it's transported into the body, it stimulates the pancreas to produce insulin. Your brain notices this increase, understands that it's busy metabolizing what you just ate, and tells you that you're less hungry. The important thing to note here is that when you consume glucose, your brain knows to tell you to stop eating when you've had enough.

Sucrose is 50% fructose and HFCS is 55% fructose (which is high compared to normal corn syrup, but pretty normal when compared to cane sugar). The remainder of each is glucose. In most cases, fructose is bad for you because of how it's processed by the body. Fructose can only be metabolized by the liver, which is not a good thing. This means a greater number of calories—about three times more than glucose—are going through your liver.

Consuming fructose changes the way your brain recognizes your intake, your brain doesn't get the message that you have not really eaten much of anything and so it thinks you're still hungry. As a result, you keep eating without necessarily realizing you're full. For example, a soda containing high amounts of fructose (which is most non-diet sodas) will do little to make you think you're full even though you're taking in large amounts of calories. This is a very, very basic look at part of how fructose is processed and doesn't even touch upon many of its other problems, but identifies the issue most people care about: fat production.

Another thing people don't realize is that sugar is actually an addictive substance. It triggers the part of the brain that deals with pleasure. It alters brain chemistry. This may be why you crave sugar when you are depressed. Hang tight and know that if we balance your sugars and alter your neurotransmitters through amino acids, it may just end the vicious cycle of your sugar cravings.

Yeast as a Hidden Cause for "Sugar Cravings"

Many times an underlying candida, or yeast, issue may be contributing to your wanting to eat sugar and carbohydrates often. If you find yourself constantly craving sugars, carbohydrates, or starches, you most likely have some sort of candida problem taking place within your body. I know from first-hand experience how tough this can be to break the cycle. Rest assured, once you kill the excess yeast in your body, you will be free of sugar cravings. It has been years since I have had any sugar or carbohydrate cravings. The study of candida can be overwhelming and seem to be a mountain of information to sort through. I have studied candida and system yeast in depth, and now understand you must kill the excess yeast to kill the sugar bug.

Oat bran and whole grain oats have been proven to lower cholesterol and stabilize blood sugar. Oats may also protect against heart disease and cancer.

Keep in mind, yeast can be a stinker to treat because it can come from hormonal imbalance, birth control pills, high stress (which causes your glucose to go high), poor diet, antibiotic use, other medications, and a whole host of other causes. It can take months or years to truly overcome this, but with patience, the right supplements, the right diet, and stress management you can control the 'sugar bug'.

I bring this topic up because your blood sugars could be out of balance from the cravings of sugar, which are actually caused by yeast. Once again, I am interested in finding the cause of problems and giving solutions to treating it.

Yeast can be treated though a good high quality probiotic supplement, candida cleanses, garlic, aloe vera, caprillic acid, and other herbs. I have specific yeast cleanses I recommend to my patients and they love the power it gives them over the dreaded sugar bug.

How to Balance Blood Sugar through Diet and Lifestyle

Most people have poor blood sugar balance; this is because most people haven't read the instructions for running a human body properly!

It is actually very easy when you know how. For your BETTER BODY, you need to balance your blood sugars and keep them balanced, as this contributes to a major part of health and longevity. My suggestion is to follow these instructions for a while and when you feel a bit more balanced then you can have 'Treats' every now and then. A healthy body can cope with the occasional high blood sugar increase.

A common misconception is that sugar gives you energy. On the contrary, a high intake of refined sugar and refined carbohydrates causes blood sugar levels to rise and fall rapidly, resulting in mood swings, tiredness, and weight gain and sugar cravings. The body just simply can't endure the roller coaster day after day. Over time, this can lead to obesity, as well as many chronic health problems like diabetes, heart disease and cancer.

The body depends on a steady and even blood sugar level. Maintaining this level will help you to feel full of energy, while at the same time stop craving sugar and stimulants, and help you to lose weight quickly - and keep it off. Steady levels of blood sugar also boost mood, memory and concentration, and reduce anxiety and depression, while cutting the risk of blood sugar-related diseases like diabetes and heart disease. Therefore the key to better health, energy and weight loss is to ensure steady blood sugar levels through simple dietary changes.

Balancing your blood sugar = more energy and feeling good!

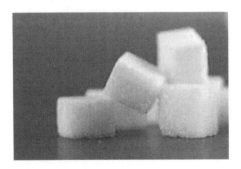

Instructions for Balancing Blood Sugar

1. Avoid sugary foods, sugar, white refined carbs, alcohol, coffee, and too much dried fruit and fruit juice.

2. Eat a substantial breakfast that contains – slow release carbohydrates (whole grains, oats, brown spelt, millet, and brown rice), proteins and fats. This combination takes a lot longer to digest and the sugars from the foods are released slowly and an insulin response is avoided.

3. Eat healthy snacks that contain some fats and proteins like nuts and seeds, avocado, whole grain spelt bread dipped in olive oil, an apple with a few fresh almonds, and a spelt cracker with avocado.

4. When you eat carbohydrates for lunch, also eat foods which contain some fats and some protein.

5. Eat a moderate evening meal with just proteins and green vegetables. This is a big key for weight loss.

6. Avoid eating carbohydrates or sugars at night, as that will raise your blood sugars and cause you to store fat during sleeping hours. Don't eat sugar, starches, or fruit from 3pm on.

7. Keep blood sugar balanced through the night by eating a snack that contains small amount of healthy green vegetable carbohydrate and a small amount of protein and fat – like seeds or nuts but in moderation.

Balancing blood sugar is important for our physical and emotional health regardless of whether you have diabetes, hypoglycemia or blood sugar management issues. A steady supply of glucose is essential to fuel peak brain functions, and therefore, low blood glucose can cause headache, irritability, anxiety and depression, dizziness, fatigue and poor endurance. Low blood sugar can also cause sugar cravings leading to erratic eating patterns.

Sugar and Your Body

Contrary to popular opinion, eating fat does not necessarily make you fat.

It's actually the way that your body stores fat that makes you gain weight. Overconsumption of carbohydrates and sugars stimulates your body's production of insulin - which is the body's fat storage hormone. Insulin lowers blood sugar levels when they are too high. However, it also causes the body to store fat.

Easier On Than Off

If you consume large amounts of starch and sugar on a frequent basis, your insulin levels will remain high. If insulin levels remain high, your fat is then locked into your fat cells. This makes it very easy to gain weight and extremely difficult to lose weight. Elevated insulin levels prevent the body from burning stored body fat for energy. Most obese patients cannot break out of this vicious cycle because they are constantly craving starchy, sugary foods throughout the day, which keeps the insulin levels elevated and prevents the body from burning these stored fats.

If you are having a craving for an unhealthy food, first do 10 pushups or jumping jacks and then decide if you still want that food. Often when you so something physical you can interrupt that craving pattern.

Exercise may not help you if you don't eat right. If you eat carbohydrates throughout the day, since the glycogen levels in your body are filled, all the excess carbohydrates will be converted to fat. The high insulin levels also tell the body not to release any of its stored fat. Therefore, you can work out for hours at a gym and still not loose fat because you are eating high amounts of carbohydrates and sugar throughout the day.

Your body will store any excess carbohydrates as fat and not release any fat that is already stored.

Low Blood Sugar

To make matters even worse, when you consume sugar or starches frequently, especially cake, candy, cookies, fruit juices, ice cream or processed white flour, you may develop low blood sugar within a few hours after eating. Symptoms of this include spaciness, shakiness, irritability, extreme fatigue, headache, sweatiness, racing heart, extreme hunger or an extreme craving for something sweet or starchy.

Other Glycemic Foods

Many high-glycemic foods are ordinary snack foods. Nearly all cereals, grains, pastas, breads, potatoes, corn, popcorn, chips, pretzels, crackers, bagels, plus other starches are high-glycemic carbohydrates. Therefore, you can certainly see why people become overweight, because these foods continue to set-off insulin release, and insulin continues to tell the body to store fat and keep it stored.

Flavored waters are growing in popularity, and their labels list water, 100 percent natural fruit flavors, and zero calories-but watch out! Most have artificial sweeteners like diet soft drinks, and those poison you. Some flavored waters are also carbonated which acidifies your body, setting you up for all kinds of disease. If you crave strawberry-flavored water, instead of buying flavored water slice a real strawberry into a glass of water. You can't beat the real thing!

Sugar also depresses your immune system by decreasing white blood cell activity. I am constantly telling my patients if they have an illness or infection, they need to get off all sugar. Sugar is like putting fuel on a fire, it will only make it worse and take longer to heal.

Diet soft drinks are no better-in fact, they're worse. Artificial sweeteners within diet drinks and other foods are highly toxic. Anytime those sweeteners get above 86 degrees, and your body temperature is normally 10 degrees hotter than that, they break down into three lethal substances. One is methanol; toxic levels of that causes blindness. An additional is formic acid; that's what poisonous insects inject into you. Why do it to

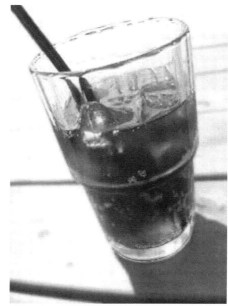

yourself? The third is cancer-causing formaldehyde. Those are not substances you want wandering around inside you.

And forget losing any pounds-with consistent use, artificial sweeteners in reality cause weight gain! Diet soft drinks have been marketed for about thirty years now, and the average weight of people in our society has gone up, not down. Clearly, we are not getting any smaller, but we are, on the average, suffering from obesity and diseases such as diabetes much more frequently.

With consistent baby steps watching what you eat and when you eat, you will rebalance your blood sugars which will yield you weight loss, increased energy, increased circulation, healthier heart, and so many other positive health improvements. Blood sugar and insulin levels being naturally brought into a healthy range is part of your BETTER BODY plan.

Chapter 6

Emotional Balance, Stress,

Positive Attitude

The third step towards a Better Body is keeping your mind in balance.

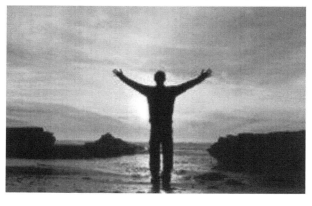 Having a positive attitude can dramatically affect how our life turns out. Our attitude will either make us or break us. Everyone has a breaking point. You must know your own limitations, your own boundaries, your standards, and where your breaking point is. If you get pushed beyond your comfort zone too often or for too

long, the results can be devastating to your health.

A positive thought actually produces different chemicals in your body, than does a negative thought. Positive thoughts heal your body, they actually promote healing. Negative thoughts will keep you sick longer; they will slow your body from healing and will make your feel like a prisoner with your own life.

Nobody has a positive attitude all the time. Everyone experiences good days, and bad days. Good months and bad months and sometimes even good years and bad years. The goal is be consistent and don't give up. Never lose hope that "this too shall pass". Many times a simple change in perception will do wonders for the soul.

For your BETTER BODY you will need to find mental "decompression" time and learn how to de-stress. Stress is one of the fastest killers known to mankind. As stress has a link to many of the top killers, such as heart disease, cancer, and diabetes. By the end of this chapter you will know some avenues you can take to slow down, decompress, and find light at the end of the tunnel.

Stress

The number one enemy of our immune system is without a doubt stress. By stress, I don't mean money troubles, problems at work, or arguments with your spouse. Those are stressors. Stress is your body's reaction to those stressors. It can stress out your body by increasing your heart rate, blood pressure, respiration, nutritional needs, and hormonal activity, all in response to a loud stimulus.

When your body goes on high alert and you're in fight-or-flight mode, physiological changes take place in your body. It's wonderful that your body helps you survive in stressful times. However, you were never designed to run on continual high alert. When you are constantly under stress or burning the candle from both ends, you are shutting down your parasympathetic nervous system, which is responsible for "rest and digest". Therefore you don't digest your food properly and you don't sleep well when you are stressed.

When your body is under stress, your body neglects your immune system because it isn't focusing on fighting cancer, infections, and traumas; it's focusing on your survival. Your body releases fight-to-flight hormones like cortisol and adrenaline to aid you in your struggle for survival.

You must free yourself from the bondage of stress and a hectic lifestyle. Stress seems to weaken the immune system and lower our resistance to illness .When people are struggling with stress they are putting extra stress on their adrenal glands.

Adrenal Fatigue

This is a topic I know first-hand. The journey of my own personal experience with phase three adrenal fatigue is what got me on the path to holistic healing and hormonal balancing. This can be a devastating condition. This can ruin relationships, cause autoimmune diseases, cancers, heart disease, nervous breakdowns, pain, or simply put, "burn out". It happens gradually. The scary thing is, it happens to the best of anyone. I had no clue it was happening. It just kind of sneaks up on you. By the time you get to phase three adrenal fatigue, it has been in the making for over 5 years.

Research has shown that being out in nature relieves mental stress and fatigue and creates a positive mood. If you are feeling stressed go for a walk in the park instead of grabbing for a candy bar.

Many times college students, new moms, competitive athletes, type A personalities, over achievers, people with chronic infections or chronic pain, long standing illnesses, business owners, financially stressed people, people who don't like their jobs and unhealthy relationships can all cause this disorder.

I have seen it as early as 14 years old and in someone 78 years old. Many times it strikes in the middle years when people notice they are constantly fatigued, easily stressed out, exhausted, easily irritable, or feel "blah" with little spark left.

The adrenal glands are tiny walnut sized glands which sit atop the kidneys. They produce hormones in response to stress and basic body functions.

They help regulate sleep, water retention, blood sugar, healing, emotions, heart rate, respiration, and every other body function. They are needed for survival.

Understanding the longer you experience stress, the further in the "hole" you go with adrenal fatigue. There are 3 different phases that occur. First, the "alarm phase" takes place, indicating something has gone wrong. Second, the "resistance phase" is the body trying to manage the stress and fatigue starts to take place. Finally, phase three is "exhaustion phase". The body has officially had it. You pushed it beyond its comfort levels. You are now living off caffeine, adrenal highs, you are "wired but tired", you can't recover, you can't lose weight, and you certainly have lost some of your peppy zest for life.

I know how painful this can be. I also know how rewarding it can be once

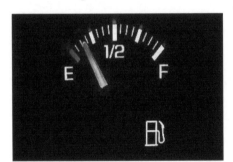

you identify you actually have adrenal fatigue and start taking steps towards fixing it. It can take months to a few years to fix this condition. It will take a change in lifestyle, diet, and the ability to rest more often.

Imagine your car is running low on fuel, you expect it to keep on running; you expect it to perform well, climb a mountain traveling through Colorado and run the air conditioner, radio, and all the other gadgets. You put a piece of duct tape over the low fuel indicator. How far do you think your car will make it? Not very far, right? The same is true for your body. You can't keep pushing it if it is already worn out. You can't expect high performance from a tired body and mind. You can deal with the "extra" irons in the fire under stress. You will eventually collapse (diseases take over), if you don't stop and listen to your body.

The neat thing about the human body that simply amazes me is it will always give us feedback. It has an inner guidance center. It knows what you need. The problem is many times we ignore these 'warning signals'. Then a few years of ignoring the warning light, we simply cannot function. We are not ourselves. At this point we simply exist. We are just hanging on for dear life. We don't have time for fun or the extra things in life; we are just trying to survive. I know because I have been there. It is not fun.

But today, I am completely free of adrenal fatigue. You can be too. You need to do a saliva test to check your cortisol levels, and your DHEA. Additionally, I would recommend a neurotransmitter test (urine test) to see how your epinephrine, norepinephrine, dopamine, serotonin, glutamate, and others are functioning. These all correlate to stress levels. If you can alter or support hormones and/or neurotransmitters you will get your life back. You will get your energy back and may be able to overcome certain diseases.

Be Your Own Health Detective

Once again, I am here to help be your human health detective. We want to know what is causing the fatigue, the weight gain, the depression, or the cancer. We want to know, how you got to the place you are at today. There is a reason. We just need to identify some possible causes.

Keep in mind, the adrenal glands deal with basic human survival. They deal with "fight or flight". They help in times of stress, whether chemical, emotional, physical, temperature, environmental, noise or illness. You will need to know how your basic survival stress glands are functioning if you expect healing, health, or happiness to occur.

Stress hormones make our bodies acidic. When this happens your body lowers body chemistry and overall health. Emotions such as happiness, optimism, and joy boost the immune system

According to Dr. Bruce Lipton, PhD Cellular Biologist, the author of Biology of Belief he states that every cell receives a "perception" of the environment as interpreted by the education brain. The human nervous system tabulates approximately four billion environmental signals per second. The primary role of it is to "read" the environment and make appropriate adjustments of growth and protection behaviors in order to ensure survival. Memory systems evolved to facilitate information handling by storing previously "learned" experiences. Memories, which represent perceptions, are scored on the basis of whether they support growth or require a protection response.

Lipton goes onto to state that cells move either forward or backward in response to thoughts. The more relevant a stimulus is to the organism's survival, the more polarized (either + or -) the resulting response. In humans, the extremes of the two polarities might appropriately be described as LOVE (+) and FEAR (-). Love fuels growth. In contrast, fear stunts growth. In fact, someone can literally be "scared to death."

Perception of environmental threats suppresses a cell's growth activities and causes it to modify its external cell structure in adopting a protection "posture." Suppressing growth mechanisms conserves valuable energy needed in exercising life-saving protection behaviors.

This work completely and totally fascinates me. Every cell reacts to our thoughts, our memories, and our environment to enable survival of the human species.

A change in attitude will take time. Many times it can take several attempts, as you may be prone to slipping back into a negative pessimistic attitude. Hang tight and know you can change. People are programmed to change. Even though you may not like it, you can do it. It takes about 3 weeks to make or break a habit. May take longer depending on how long habits or attitudes have been entrenched. Attitudes are known to become a habit.

Transition your "inner talk" to be positive and hopeful. Be filled with faith. Know that you deserve a happy life. Know that God wants you to have a happy life. Know that your body is made in the image and likeness of God. You are dwelling in His Temple. Be kind with your thoughts. Be kind to your body.

The Sum of You

Don't try to quit all your bad habits at once; the shock will be too much for you to handle. Do a slow, steady easy does it attitude. Have a coach. Read books. Watch and learn from others who are where you want to be. YOU WILL BECOME THE SUM TOTAL OF the books you read, the music you listen to, the TV shows you watch, the people you hang out with, and the habits you develop. So are you on the constructive or destructive path? Are you growing or shrinking? Are you inspiring or draining? Are you living or dying? It's your choice. You are the artist of your canvas of life.

There is truth to the statement "who you hang around, is who you become". I once heard a statement that you will eventually become the sum total of the 5 people you hang around the most. So think about it, are your hanging around healthy or unhealthy people? Are you hanging around financially secure people or broke people? Are you hanging around married or divorced people? Are you hanging around drinkers or non-drinkers? You will become many times who you associate with.

Surround yourself with positive uplifting people, books, music, CD's, audios, and activities. Learn to incorporate affirmations daily. Start your day with positive statements before you even get out of bed. Go to bed each night with deep breaths, prayers, gratitude, and positive thoughts. Shut your mind off from negative news before bed. Listen to soft relaxing music. Use lavender aroma therapy.

Using Affirmations or Positive "inner talk"

The words we speak on a daily basis are who we ultimately become. If you want a better body, you must start thinking and speaking differently. Just as it states in the Bible, what is in a man's heart, comes out through his words.

Use the following statements at least twice daily: once each morning and once before falling asleep.

- I love life. Life loves me.
- I am learning to be comfortable in my own body.
- I am grateful for the good things in my life.
- My day goes smooth and effortless.
- I am a calm, centered person.
- Everything I do brings me joy.
- It is a joy to speak to myself in kind and loving ways.
- I sleep well at night. I wake up refreshed.
- The more I love my body, the healthier I feel.
- I am healthy, wealthy, and wise!
- I release negative incidents with love, it is over and done.
- Only good experiences lie before me.
- I release all drama from my life and now get energy from peace.

- I am worthy of abundance.
- I trust Life to take care of me.
- I love my family. And my family loves me.
- I create happy, healthy relationships all around me.
- I attract loving people into my life.
- I am smart and resourceful.
- I have plenty of time each day to get everything done.

Here are Some Additional Positive Affirmations You May Want to Try for the Ultimate Mental Shift in Health.

- My body has 'inner intelligence' and knows how to heal.
- My body wants to heal and is always working towards health.
- I make wise lifestyle choices every day to help my body in the healing process.
- I am attracting health and happiness into my life daily.
- I am living a balanced lifestyle.
- I hydrate my body and brain with at least 6-8 glasses of pure fresh water daily.
- I eat only healthy, wholesome foods. I eat vibrant colored fruits and vegetables. I eat mainly 'white' meats and fish.
- I avoid all processed or prepackaged foods, as I know they are unhealthy for my body.
- I am eliminating all sugar, soda, sweets, and candy from my diet.
- I enjoy taking 10 slow deep breaths before going to sleep at night.
- I give myself permission to sleep restfully each night.
- I respect my body.
- I love to be energized.
- I deserve to live a long, healthy, active life.
- I understand healing takes time. I am patient during my healing process.
- I am realistic with my goals and expectations of myself.
- I love taking time daily to slooooow down and relax. I am simplifying my life.
- I receive love and give love easily.

- Each day I am getting better and better.
- I am learning to be a happier and more grateful person.
- I avoid excessive alcohol and caffeine.
- I trust the decisions I make. I trust my intuition or 'inner voice'.
- I deserve to be happy.
- I am worthy of improving my health and well-being.
- I am forgiving. I can forgive 'hurts' from my past.
- I expect healing.
- I can follow directions and advice from my doctor.
- I give myself permission to say 'no' at times.
- I accept and love myself.
- I laugh often, as I realize "laughter is the best medicine". I am trying to enjoy the life I was given.
- I can remain calm. I know that "this too shall pass".
- I remind myself daily to try to help others and be kind to others. For it is in "giving that we receive".

When changing your lifestyle habits from unhealthy habits to healthy habits, focus on your progress not on perfection.

Remember, we are a three-part being: body, soul and spirit. For overall health and well-being you have to look a little deeper than the skin.

You are in the process of achieving a better body; you are ready to transform your life. Part of this equation is you must be aware of your boundaries and your limitations. You must listen to your body. When you are over-extending yourself, you must pull back or you will pay the consequences. The time is now for you to realize what is happening on the inside of your body. It can't survive "high alert" for extended periods of time.

Serotonin is a neurotransmitter that seems to reduce anxiety as it produces satiety. Other neurotransmitters such as dopamine, norepinephrine, and endorphins can also affect our feelings of satiety and anxiety. There are now more than one hundred known neurotransmitters, and many more of them may affect mood in the response to food in ways that are just beginning to be researched and understood.

I have been using a company where we can use a simple urine test to evaluate the levels of your neurotransmitters in your brain. If you are too high in the "excitatory" neurotransmitters, you will feel overly anxious or "ramped up", unable to relax. At the same time, if you low in your "inhibitory" neurotransmitters, this could explain why you are sluggish, unmotivated, depressed, and easily irritated.

Once I look to see where your highs and lows are, we can use amino acids to balance the neurotransmitters out. Amino acids are the precursors to the neurotransmitters in the brain. It makes more sense to help people balance out their brain chemistry through natural amino acids, rather than using pharmaceutical drugs, such as anti-depressant drugs..

Stress Busting Techniques

- **Identify stressors**. Each day sit down and reevaluate what made you tense. Think back to all the "irons in the fire" for that day. You can't fight off stress if you don't take time to know what is causing it.
- **Eliminate unnecessary commitments**. Today more than ever, the schedules are out of control. With sports, work, organizations, and family obligations. Something may have to give. Give yourself permission to find time to slow down and not be involved in every organization or club. Say no occasionally.
- **Procrastination**. This gets the best of us. But if you do a little each day from your "to do list", soon enough it will be shrinking down to a manageable list. The key is to do it as it comes up if possible.
- **Disorganization**. The more organized you feel, the less stress you will have. When people are organized they feel in control of their surroundings.
- **Late**. If you have to, get up 15 minutes earlier each morning. If you need to, set a timer to help you get out of the door on time. Running late makes you feel tense and rushed, which makes your body produce lots of stress hormones, leading to more stress.
- **Controlling**. The more in control you are, the less stress you will have. People who have things under control typically are relaxed and organized. Start controlling your money management, your eating habits, your exercise habits, and your attitude. Once you do this, you will feel full of energy and have a great outlook.

- **Multitasking**. This leads to stress because you can't focus on several things at once and do a good job at all of them. You really can only do one thing at a time well. So slow down, and just focus on one project at a time.
- **Eliminate energy drains**. We all know people or environments that "suck our energy". Try really hard to avoid these people or situations. Being around this will only make you exhausted and irritable.
- **Avoid difficult people**. Identify who these people are and put a mental shield around yourself when you are near these people. Realize they are the ones who need help, most likely not you. You are only doing the best you can when around these people. Pray for them.
- **Simplify life.** The quicker you simplify and don't over complicate things, the happier you will be. You need to take time and look at the areas of your life that can be simplified. Maybe you can slow down your schedule, maybe you can reduce your spending habits, or better yet maybe you could hire it done so you can relax a bit more.

In addition to the lifestyle changes mentioned above try to aim for several of the stress reducing techniques daily to achieve your BETTER BODY. You will live a longer more enjoyable life if you control your stress levels. At the core of most diseases there is a contributing factor of stress (physical, chemical, financial, emotional, social, hormonal, or other) that plays a role in the destruction of your health.

Holistic Treatment Views

- Chiropractic adjustments reduce tension on the nervous system and are highly affective for stress releasing.
- Acupuncture stimulates the body's own calming mechanism. I have many patients who use acupuncture as their first line of stress relief because it works instantly.
- Have your adrenal glands checked through saliva testing. Adrenals actually are your stress glands and can be evaluated how well they are working. We can look at DHEA and cortisol levels to see really how stressed you are, and in what 'stage' of stress you are in.

- Take minerals. Magnesium is mother nature's miracle mineral for stress reduction.
- Take B-vitamins, it help with stress.
- Deep breath, slow deep belly breaths. 5-10 when you are highly stressed. Deep slow breaths also alkalize the body's chemistry.
- Use your affirmations, find yourself an "anchoring positive word or phrase" such as: "calm", or my favorite is "this too shall pass"
- Prayer always helps to calm stress.
- Exercise can reduce stress by up to 60%.
- Eat high protein snacks; protein is the precursors to neurotransmitters, which makes your serotonin and happy brain chemicals.
- Eat healthy fats, such as nuts or avocados. They help with brain function.
- Avoid sugars and junk foods; it only makes you more toxic, leaving you to feel worse.
- Avoid caffeine, especially when stress is high. Caffeine will only stimulate you more.
- Take a hot bubble bath, as this reduces cortisol levels.
- Listen to relaxing music.
- Use aromatherapy, such as lavender.
- Listen to happy upbeat music to get you to your "happy spot".
- Take a nap, stress requires a lot of work. Rest will rejuvenate.
- Drink hot decaffeinated green tea, it releases an amino acid to increase brain calming activity.
- Stay hydrated. If you are dehydrated you will not handle stress as efficiently.
- Keep your hormones balanced! Imbalanced hormones have a lot to do with your stress levels. Typically natural progesterone is a wonderful natural "calming hormone". Do not deal with hormones on your own; as if you do not need them, you should not use them.
- Consume a whey protein shake to boost serotonin and neurotransmitters.
- Get to sleep earlier.

- Stay hydrated.

To achieve your better body transformation, now is as good of a time as ever to start saying no to extra projects. You need to start doing some deep breathing daily to reduce the stress off your diaphragm region. Make daily affirmations a daily activity, this will allow you to feel more inspired and bring your confidence levels up. Identify how much protein you are eating and start eating more. If you eat more protein and eat healthy fats, such as nuts and avocados you will feel mentally stronger, as high protein foods are precursors to serotonin and other neurotransmitters. Staying hydrated with clean fresh water will keep your brain working at its best. Finally, evaluating your hormones and adrenal functions, as this will allow for your stress handling glands to have a fight chance to help you deal with stress. If your hormones are out of balance you will never feel healthy. You can do this. Just take small baby steps and soon you will be experiencing your happy self.

Chapter 7

Hormones:

The Key to Longevity and Sanity

The fourth step towards a Better Body is keeping the hormones balanced.

Hormones are biochemical compounds produced by various organs or glands of the body. Hormones are essential to life function. Without hormones, we really cannot survive. They control most aspects of all of our bodily processes. Our hormones control our brain function, our bone

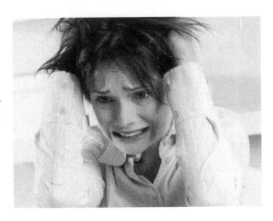

functions, our reproductivity, our sex drive and so many other functions.

Our hormones work together. For instance, estrogen and progesterone are both steroid hormones that are dependent on each other. Cortisol and DHEA are adrenal hormones that have just such a relationship. Balance is the key to proper hormone function and therefore, bodily function. When hormones become imbalanced, problems are next in line to come into the picture. The "system of checks and balances" of our endocrine system will normally respond in an opposite direction. If one hormone goes up, the partner hormone will fall to keep things balanced. Leaving you to feeling way "out of balance".

Signs and Symptoms of Hormonal Imbalance

- Depression
- Fatigue
- Bloating/ Gas
- Thinning hair/ hair loss
- Weight gain
- "Muffin Top"/ Middle "spare tire"
- Hot flashes/ night sweats
- Headaches
- Wrinkles
- Low sex drive
- Insomnia
- Heart problems/ palpitations
- Feeling 'blah', lack of joy
- High stress levels
- Acne/ skin problems
- Pain and joint stiffness
- Bleeding gums
- Constipation
- These are just a few, plenty more

Testing Your Hormones

When hormone imbalance is suspected, it is vitally important to properly test your hormone levels. Without testing, it is impossible to know what is going on with your hormones. Treating in such a manner is absolutely crazy practice. However, it happens all of the time. Doctors prescribe birth control pills, give hormone creams, and/or give injections or patches every day. All without testing to see what the patient's true hormone levels are at that time. By evaluating results, and treating properly, great results and a return of health and happiness will follow testing and treatment. Testing is a powerful step in the healing process of hormones. Testing allows us to look at the whole picture of a person's physical and mental well-being.

Private Testing

Many women and men would like to feel better but are embarrassed to talk about their hormones, sex life, or moods. Today you can have a detailed evaluation of all your hormones even if your family medical doctor does not believe your problems could be hormone related. To test your hormones, you will request a kit to be mailed to you. Once your kit comes in the mail, you collect your saliva (spit) in 4 colored tubes, according to the time of the day. You fill out a small amount of paper work and then mail the samples in on a pre-addressed UPS label. If you are cycling woman who still gets her period, you will need to take the test days 19-21 of your cycle. If you have had a hysterectomy, in menopause or have an irregular cycle you can collect your samples anytime. Men can do samples any day. It is easy to do and very discrete. Results will come back to the doctor and we will call you to discuss your results.

Hormonal Imbalance Consequences

Today men and women are suffering needlessly. Their families are falling apart and moods are crumbling all because of hormonal imbalances. Young gals are wanting to start a family and wondering why they can't conceive. An aging woman wonders why she can't remember anything. A man in his fifties has had his first heart attack and is constantly irritable and fatigued. These are all hormonal imbalances. Hormone imbalance is a true epidemic in our country. The average American female and male over 35 years of age suffers from some form of hormonal imbalance. High stress, bad diets, foreign hormones added to foods, lack of exercise all contribute to the imbalances. The symptoms many times are gradual and sneak up over years. It strikes the best of anyone. Nobody is discriminated against when it comes to hormones.

It becomes a vicious cycle that slowly robs you of your energy, your vitality and your life and lifestyle. It is very hard to get your hormones back in balance by yourself. You really should have your hormones evaluated for your base lines. You will need to find a holistic doctor or contact my office for help.

How Do Your Hormones Get Out of Balance?

The longer you have suffered, the longer it may take to rebalance. There are many situations and events that contribute to your imbalances. Overwork, physical and mental overstrain, sleep deprivation, noise pollution, late hours, surgery, medications, injuries, inflammation, pain, toxicity, ingestion of chemicals, poor diet filled with packaged and processed non-nutritive foods, electromagnetic fields, poor digestion, blood sugar issues, environmental xenohormones, allergies, and the list goes on and on.

Patients experiencing a majority of these symptoms most likely will benefit from natural hormone replacement. The most effective way to assess hormone status is to test saliva for the appropriate hormone levels. Saliva is the best method for testing "functional" tissue levels of hormones.

I want women to know that the estrogen levels drop by approximately 40% at menopause while progesterone levels plummet by approximately 90% from premenopausal levels. It is the relative loss of progesterone that causes the majority of symptoms termed estrogen dominance. The Progesterone/Estradiol (Pg/E2) reference ranges are optimal ranges determined by Dr. John Lee. While they are not physiological ranges, they are optimal values for the protection of the breasts, heart and bones in women, and the prostate in men.

Contrary to popular belief, **Menopause is not simply the result of estrogen deficiency**; although, estrogen levels do decline during the latter phases of a woman's reproductive cycle. Estrogen levels drop by approximately 40% at menopause while progesterone levels plummet to approximately 90% of the pre-menopausal levels. **It is the relative loss of progesterone that causes the majority of symptoms.** The disproportionate loss of progesterone begins in the latter stages of a woman's reproductive cycle, while unbeknownst to her; the luteal phase of the menstrual cycle begins to malfunction. The malfunction is initiated when the remnant tissue of the follicle (corpus luteum), the primary source of progesterone, begins to lose its functional capacity. By approximately age 35, many of these follicles fail to develop creating a relative progesterone deficiency. As a result, ovulation does not always occur and progesterone levels steadily decline. It is during this period that a relative progesterone deficiency, or what has become known as **Estrogen Dominance**, develops.

The most effective way to assess hormone status is to test saliva for the appropriate hormone levels. The reason that saliva is the best method of testing is that "active" tissue levels are measured, opposed to serum testing in which essentially measures the "inactive" levels.

Hormonal Balancing for Women

Hormonal balancing is a **personal choice** for each woman. You are each **created differently**, from different genetic backgrounds, lifestyles, ways you handle stress, diets, relationships, and your personal needs.

What a gift to know that **there is** help in this area. If you can balance your hormones you literally will change your attitude, your body, your sleep habits, your outlook, your performance, and your energy levels.

This topic is intimidating not only to you, the consumer; but also many doctors or health care professionals. You must take charge of your own body and emotions through learning and becoming educated in this topic.

Start learning more! **Learn the values of your hormones.** Learn and become an active participant, don't be passive. If there were ever one topic to not be passive in, this is it! This can be the difference in how you age, what you look like, how you act, and your future health's fate. The pendulum has swung for women's health concerns.

80% of women experience hormonal imbalances. There are too many demands of us and not enough support. Simply put, God did not create us to work outside the home, run the kids to several different activities, eat all the junk we eat, take care of everyone else's problems, go to all the organizations, clubs, and meetings we go to, go home and do everything we have to do at home for everyone else, or be sedentary .So...........ladies, many of us are doing more than we can handle; not eating the right foods that nourish our bodies, don't take enough time for us, not moving enough, don't relax enough, and we are bombarded with endocrine disruptors. Be prepared to read some of the most important information as a woman living in a challenging time of history. **85% of women can receive therapeutic balancing of hormones through diet, lifestyle change, medical grade nutritional supplements, and bio-identical progesterone cream.**

Hormones are named after the Greek "hormao" ("I stir up"). Some say that it is from the Greek "hormon", meaning "to urge on" from "horme", meaning "impulse". Hormones were not discovered until the early 20th century. Over 50 have been identified; and new ones are still being discovered.

"So many women are afraid to take herbal remedies because they're uncertain about safety. They think that because a pharmaceutical drug has been studied in a laboratory, regulated by the FDA and prescribed by a doctor, it has to be safe. But the truth is that conventional medicine is responsible for 255,000 deaths per year in the United States, and almost half of those are from adverse reactions to prescription drugs." Dr. Marcelle Pick, OB/GYN.

Phytotherapy is the use of plants, either in whole food form or in the form of standardized extracts and supplements, for healing purposes. Its roots trace all the back to the beginning of time and still stands strong in much of the world today. It is much gentler on our bodies than pharmaceutical medications. They are used to prevent conditions and treat conditions.

The National Cancer Institute currently defines the word "phytoestrogen" as an estrogen-like substance found in some plants and plant products. They also state that phytoestrogens may have anti-cancer effects.

"Botanical therapies for menopause symptoms are taking an increasingly important role. Many women are determined to utilize therapies that are herbal or nutritional, natural hormones, or lower dose hormones in combination with botanicals, in order to create a risk to benefit ration that they feel comfortable with." Dr. Hudson, Women's Health Specialist at Women to Women.

Become an advocate to other women that there are answers. Women are smart today. We are educating ourselves. We are searching for answers. We want to be beautiful. We want to feel in control of our bodies. We want to age gracefully. Now days, women are gaining professional degrees, then starting families in their forties. You just need to make a priority to find **a healthy balanced lifestyle to keep your hormones happy.**

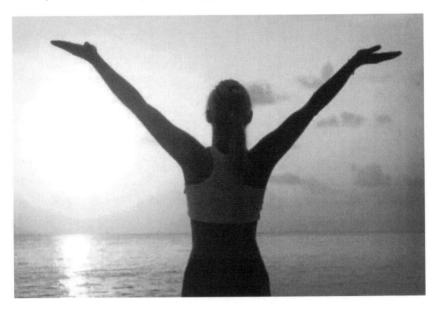

Phases of the Female Maturation Process

Normal cycle: 28-30 days in length. Day 1-14 follicular phase (estrogen is more predominant), Day 15-30 Luteal Phase (progesterone predominantly)

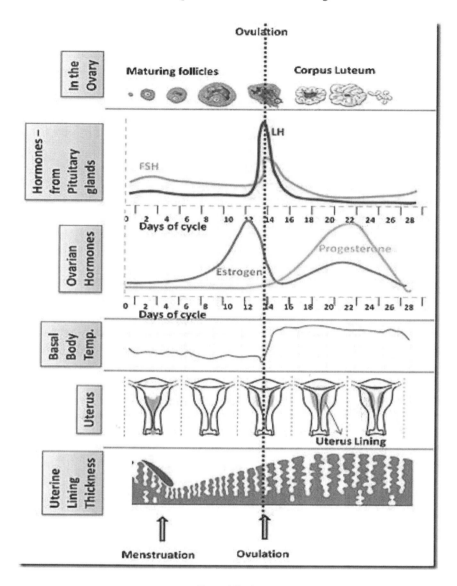

Normal Cycle

Perimenopause: A time period leading up to menopause, may last from 5-15 years.

Menopause: The time period when a woman has not had a period for longer than a year.

Xenohormones

Most of you will have never heard of this word. Most of you will not know how dangerous common products can be to your reproductive health. The word "XENO" means "foreign". And this term describes chemicals that are man-made and foreign to the body, and which mimic or block normal hormone function.

- Increase in reproductive-site cancers in women and men
- Decreased fertility in both sexes
- Decreased sperm count in males (human and animals)
- Low testosterone levels
- Increased incidence of undescended testicles
- Increasing PMS / fertility problems in women

Technology and the evolution of modern medicine have never been better. Nevertheless, people are getting fatter as well as sicker than ever before with growing rates of diabetes, obesity, cancer, and infertility among men, women, & children.

Countless men & women are dealing with all kinds of hormone based issues. Something is critically wrong with our existing level of hormonal wellbeing. What is to blame?

The over dependence on highly prepared, chemically-laden industry based goods and foodstuffs seems to be the chief culprit. Xenoestrogens are artificially made compounds produced by industry. These differ chemically from archiestrogens (naturally occurring) produced by living organisms.

Xenoestrogens mimic the effects of authentic estrogen and interact with cellular receptor sites. This process contributes to an estrogen surplus and blocks the effects of authentic estrogen. To make matters worse, these endocrine disruptors lodge in fat cells where they are resistant to breakdown. Several of these chemicals will act in a synergistic effect when combined with other endocrine disrupters. This synergistic process greatly enhances their effects inside the body causing major problems at the cellular level.

In the past 60 years over 87,000 new chemicals have been introduced into our food, water, air supply. Up until this, the body only had its own hormones or plant hormones to worry about. "Is it in the water? It sure does make you wonder. I would say YES.

There have been dozens of these chemicals routinely found in human tissues, the blood stream and even human breast milk. ***The Major concern is they ACCUMULATE! That's the real problem. Nobody has studied the synergistic effect of these.*** The endocrine system responds to extremely tiny levels of chemicals. It is the most sensitive system of the body. Larger or smaller amounts of chemicals activate the endocrine system in different ways. Many chemicals can exert multiple hormone disruptor effects. Endocrine disruptors affect well-being, cognition, thyroid, metabolism, digestion, and hormonal imbalances.

Some of the common Hormone disruptors are: Pesticides, herbicides, insecticides. Plastics. Plasticizers ("thalates") cling wraps, Bisphenol A (plastic), pharmaceuticals, Dioxins, chlorines, PVC, detergents: cosmetics, hair products, soaps, shaving cream, and nail polish.

Many people and scientist now think that we are the guinea pigs in the largest uncontrollable science experiment in history. No one knows the long term effects of all these endocrine disruptors. Many experts and health providers are speculating an increase in childhood cancers, infertility, learning disabilities, autism, chemical sensitivities, even cancers.

Holistic options to increase your chances of protecting your body from most forms of Cancer

- Become a health advocate. Become educated!
- Correct and eliminate all estrogen dominance
- Minimize Xenohormone exposure
- Address risk factors
- Exercise 5 days a week.
- Consider emotional psychological factors
- Strengthen adrenal function
- Strengthen immune function
- Alkalize the body pH
- Become informed about the politics of the Breast Cancer Industry
- Mediterranean type diets are best for cancer prevention.

- Eat a diet high in fiber, vegetables, and fruit.

To help you feel your best and achieve your BETTER BODY, Detoxification Programs help to eliminate excess build up in system. Additionally, learning about hormones, bio-identical treatments, natural weight loss systems are the best bet to protect your present and future health.

Ways to Protect Your Body from Hormonal Imbalances

- Lessen the usage of endocrine disruptors as much as possible. Get off all oral contraceptives, hormone creams, in addition to hormone based prescription medications, and so forth. You should consult your alternative health practitioner or open-minded medical professional about this and weaning stages may well be essential.

- Even out Your Blood Sugar. Unstable blood sugar causes enhanced fat storage, decreased cellular detoxification and hormone signaling. A healing eating plan is essential for quick efficient blood sugar stabilization.

- Do quarterly detoxes. Start by cleansing the liver & gallbladder so they can effectively transport surplus estrogen out of the system. Enrich your estrogen metabolism with key nutrients & herbs. Lastly, sustain the pituitary gland with plenty rest, movement, along with nutritional components. Detoxing helps with hormonal imbalance

- Maximize your nervous system. Get under regular chiropractic care. Be sure that the brain-body pathway is clear and free of interference. This maximizes interior restoration mechanisms. With a strong nervous system, the glands and tissues are capable to self-detoxify and get rid of toxic chemical substances. Forward head posture and loss of the natural curve in the neck dramatically have an effect on this self-detoxification process.

- Great intensity exercise opens detoxification pathways (sweating), enhances cellular oxygenation, and stabilizes blood sugar, along with promoting reparative hormones among other things. Also, it enables the body to lose fat more effectively and to metabolize excess estrogen molecules.

- Acupuncture has been gained much popularity in the past decade with treating hormonal problems, infertility, hot flashes, stress and many other hormone related symptoms. Treatments are very effective.

- Eating low fat, Mediterranean type diets, low glycemic index foods

- Have your hormones evaluated once a year. Use ONLY bio-identical hormone replacements if you need any.

- Consume Flaxseed/ oil

- Indole -3- carbinole taken as a supplement (helps produce estrogen) (protective)

- Indole 3 Carbinol is found in cruciferous vegetables.

- High protein diet, mainly fish, chickens, low fats

- Omega fatty acids

- B6, 12 and folate

- Black Cohosh, Red Clover, Chastetree, Passionflower, Ashwagandha, Wild Yam, Soy are all herbs for menopausal relief. Don't take herbs and drugs in the same sitting. Know contraindications before taking herbs with drugs.

- Learn about proper digestion aids to help with absorption of your nutrients and foods.

- Learn about and address adrenal fatigue (stress management)

- Detoxification (don't assume on your own, you must know about this), many of the hormones are processed through the liver. So do liver cleanses.

- Overcome constipation: It gets rid of the toxins. (Probiotics, food changes, water, fiber, medications, detoxing)

- Stress management, adrenal support to avoid adrenal fatigue

- Learn all you can about natural progesterone or estrogen therapy and how to cycle it. (Since it is natural the body excretes it easily and has an adaptogenic effect)

- Learn ways to increase serotonin naturally.......satisfaction center. (protein-tryptophan, amino acids, certain foods, meditative activity, enjoyable hobbies, get outdoors 30 minutes per day, sleep cycles, B vitamins, exercise, anything that makes you feel good)

- Have patience and retest every three months in the beginning. Sometimes it can take 3-4 switches of dosages to get it right. Don't assume it is not working.

"As a species, we`re on a fast track to extinction. In the past few decades, men have lost 50% of their sperm count and within only one generation, the average man's sperm count and testosterone have dropped by 20%. Women are no better. Staggering statistics illustrate that most women today are suffering from female disorders and three out of ten women between the ages of 35 to 60 will develop breast cancer." Ori Hofmekler, author of The Anti-Estrogenic Diet.

Chapter 8

Environmental and Other Toxins

Another step in Holistic Health and healing must be detoxifying from your exposure to toxic substances, chemicals, foods, medications, beverages, negative thoughts, radiation, constant electromagnetic pollution, poor air quality, and so many other forms of toxic ingestion. You will achieve a cleaner, healthier body which will carry you well into your golden years feeling rejuvenated, flexible, pain-free, full of joy, and aging gracefully. The more you know and understand how important this step in your transformation, the more you will appreciate this step in your key to health!

Detoxification Options

When you feel congested or toxic, it is always wise to take steps toward detoxifying, including drinking plenty of water, getting extra sleep, eating right, exercising, taking proper nutrients and utilizing a steam or sauna. Toxins must be mobilized, bound, and removed for good results.

Mobilization without sufficient binding may cause or increase "detox symptoms"; make sure enough binding power is being supplied. Detoxification, depending on the individual and severity of toxic load, can vary from a protocol of adding an herbal supplement for detoxification to the diet.

How Does the Body Remove Toxic Substances?

A person's ability to remove or detoxify toxins is a primary factor in susceptibility to toxin-related conditions. In order to remove (excrete) the wide variety of toxins, the body has a complex system that converts them into non-toxic molecules for removal. This complex system occurs in a two-phase process (Phase I and Phase II liver detoxification). Maintaining balance between phase I and phase II liver detoxification is critical, or you will get overloaded with toxins. The majority of detoxification occurs in the liver, however all tissues have some ability to detoxify, including the intestines, skin, and lungs.

Furthermore, a significant side effect of all this metabolic activity is the production of free radicals as the toxins are transformed; resulting in oxidative stress (this is what makes us age or break down faster). Nutrients that help protect us from oxidative stress include vitamins C and E, zinc, selenium, and copper.

Common Clinical Symptoms & Conditions

Associated With Environmental Toxins

- Headaches
- Fertility problems
- Multiple Chemical Sensitivities
- Learning Disorders
- Fibromyalgia
- Mood Swings
- Memory Loss
- Tinnitus/ Sinus
- Fatigue/ Weight gain
- Abnormal Pregnancy outcomes

- Mineral imbalances
- Depression
- Yeast infections
- Chronic Fatigue Syndrome
- Contact Dermatitis
- Parkinson's Disease
- Muscle Weakness
- Cancer
- Panic Attacks
- Chronic immune System issues

The most significant components of food that play the largest role in weight gain and obesity are foods additives, chemicals, and food processing techniques! It's not the food itself; it's not really the calories, the amount of fat, the amount of carbohydrates, sodium, glycemic index level, or proteins.

It's how food is processed and the man-made chemicals and additives in the food that actually cause weight gain and obesity. These include bovine growth hormone and antibiotics injected into meat, poultry, and dairy products, flavor enhancers, such as monosodium glutamate, artificial sweeteners such as NutraSweet (aspartame) and Splenda (sucralose). This also includes man-made sugars such as high fructose corn syrup, corn syrup, dextrose, sucrose, fructose, highly refined white sugar, processed molasses, processed honey, malto dextrin, etc., plus the over 15,000 chemicals that routinely added to virtually every product you buy, including conventionally grown fruits and vegetables.

> Dyes and chemicals used to flavor and preserve junk food, require a lot of extra vitamins and minerals from the body just to metabolize and detoxify them. Because junk food has no nutrients in it, the body must use its precious stores of nutrients to digest junk food.

Man-made trans fats such as hydrogenated or partially hydrogenated oils cause weight gain and obesity. Additionally, food processing techniques such as pasteurization, which is now done on virtually every product in a bottle or carton, homogenization, and irradiation (which is done to over 50% of all food products sold in America) all cause weight gain.

Saunas for Detoxification

Saunas are great for flushing out the toxins that build up in your body's fat cells. Your kidneys are detoxification powerhouses, and the intense sweating you can enjoy while spending time in a sauna can clear out about one-third of the toxic material that your kidneys remove from your bloodstream.

Multiple studies have shown that saunas are effective in removing solvents, organic chemicals, PCBs, pharmaceuticals, and heavy metal toxins from the human body.

The health benefits of using a sauna don't stop at detoxification, although they do fit in with the core values of a detoxified lifestyle. For instance, the high temperatures of a sauna can give your immune system a boost. The number of white blood cells that fight infections increases as much as 58 percent with the levels of increased temperature you get in a sauna.

Exercise for Detoxification

Among of the many benefits of exercise which is becoming popular nowadays is that it helps our body detoxify. Yes, you heard it right. Body detoxification means the removal of toxins or cleansing of vital organs in the body. Toxins do not necessarily means it come from drugs or alcohol, but toxins we get from our diet, pollution, and exposure from industrial solvents and other industrial chemicals as well.

How does exercise helps our body detoxifies? Exercise hastens body detoxification process. It keeps our body moving and speeds up the blood circulation. The response of our body every time we engage in exercise is to take in enough oxygen. Oxygen is essential to make our cells function, and among its function is to remove toxins.

How can we help our body detoxifies? We can flush out toxins in the form of sweat, exhalation and urine. When you exercise you sweat a lot, thus it can remove your body toxins. This is another reason why sedentary lifestyle must be avoided.

Lymphatic brushing for Detoxification

The lymph system helps regulate and control illnesses in your body by removing debris or toxins. The lymph system is a very intricate series of lymph nodes, lymph ducts, lymphoid organs, and lymphatic tissues. The lymph capillaries and lymph vessels produce and transport lymph fluid or toxic fluid from tissues to your circulatory system. When the lymph system is flowing smoothly toxins will be released from your body and your overall health will be improved.

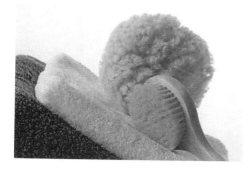

Lymphatic Body Brushing, also known as Dry Skin Brushing, is an easy technique to learn and the health benefits are spectacular. The technique begins by using a Natural Bristle Brush to lightly brush the skin beginning with the feet and then moving upwards, in the direction of the heart.

Dry brushing supports skin renewal, stimulates the lymphatic system (which positively affects the nervous, immune, and digestive systems), aids in removal of accumulated toxins, and brightens the spirit, giving your body and mind a fresh glow. As the name implies, it is practiced when the skin is dry, before bathing or applying oil or lotion. This promotes exfoliation, skin renewal and revitalization, and the stimulation of the lymphatic and nervous systems beneath the skin. Before a bath or shower is a delightful time to include dry brushing in your daily routine, especially since the subsequent immersion in water can support the removal of dead skin and continue the detoxification process.

Soda Baths for Detoxification

More than just soothing, a detox bath helps the body cleanse through its largest organ - the skin.

This is not just taking a bath for removing dirt and odors but rather a deep cleansing process that draws toxins out of the body through the sweat glands. Any of the elements can be helpful on its own.

For example, the hot water stimulates healthy perspiration and allows your body temperature to rise then fall, boosting melatonin production for swift and blissful sleep. But if your health situation allows and you have all the ingredients, the combination provides a special kind of magic.

Obviously taking a bath with this kind of heat and purpose is not for everyone. Check with your healthcare provider especially if you have a chronic heart, skin, or neurologic condition.

Detox Bath Recipe

Ingredients

1 c. Epsom salt	1 c. sea salt
1 c. baking soda	1/2 c. grated fresh ginger*

Directions

Grab a washcloth for sponging off and a glass of water (no ice) to rehydrate yourself. Begin filling your tub with comfortably hot water, then add all the ingredients and stir. Climb into the tub and soak 20-30 minutes, adding more cold or hot water if needed. Towel dry then get dressed for bed. Expect lots of perspiration, even an hour or more after your bath. You may want to set a glass of water by your bed in case you wake up thirsty.

* Can substitute 4 capsules ginger supplement or 1 teaspoon ground ginger.

The detox bath can be especially powerful when you are coming down with a cold or flu. Nothing like sweating out the toxins - and a good night's sleep - to give your body the winning edge.

Lemon Water for Detoxification

<u>Benefits of Lemon Water</u>

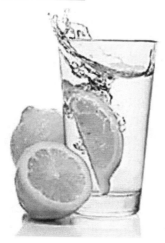

<u>Better Digestion</u>: Lemon juice stimulates saliva and the production of digestive enzymes in the stomach for better nutrient absorption. The citric acid helps relieve gas and constipation and can even destroy intestinal worms.

<u>Healthy pH Level</u>: Don't let the high citric acid content and tart flavor fool you. Lemon juice is actually a wonderful alkalizer for the body. Being overly acidic is a common problem and results in a weakened fatigued body which is prone to disease. If you are tired, achy, and sick all the time, you likely have chronically low pH. Whole diet plans have been crafted to reverse this condition, but daily lemon water is an easy step in the right direction. To monitor your baseline pH level, using a saliva test strip before drinking lemon water is most accurate.)

<u>Natural Diuretic</u>: Lemon juice is a natural diuretic, which means it increases urine flow to encourage proper water balance in the body and cleanse the kidneys. Lemon juice even helps dissolve kidney stones over time.

<u>Less Mucus</u>: Some foods encourage mucus production, such as milk products. But lemon has the opposite effect and actually dissolves mucus throughout the body. Try it next time you have sinus congestion. You may even feel the mucus melting away.

<u>Increased Fat Metabolism</u>: Lemon has a cleansing and stimulating effect on the liver and liquefies bile for better fat metabolism. Lemon juice is high in citric acid and vitamins B12 and B3, which help break down fat cells.

<u>Balanced Blood Sugar</u>: Lemon juice is a good source of bioflavonoids, especially quercetin. Quercetin is known to stimulate insulin production and help regulate blood sugar levels, which makes you feel better physically and emotionally. Balanced blood sugar also reduces cravings and encourages healthy weight loss.

<u>Stronger Immune System</u>: The vitamin C and quercetin in lemon juice promote healthy immune function, and its strong antiseptic and germicidal qualities naturally ward off disease. Lemon juice also helps dissolve uric acid and other toxins.

The bottom line is with all the toxins we are bombarded with in the environment, foods, beauty products, water, and medication, if you want longevity and a better body, you must start now detoxifying your body. You have to start taking action with certain herbs, exercise regimens, lemon water and other means of cleansing. This takes the burden off your cells, your liver and your lungs allowing you to gain energy and live longer.

Even though we are surrounded by toxins, you can avoid certain diseases and heal conditions you have by detoxing your lifestyle, your body, and reduce environmental exposures. Not only will you live longer, you will ensure the genetic make-up of your family heritage line. By using this information you are now empowered to make informed decisions in protecting yourself and your family from the toxins we come across in our daily lives.

Chapter 9

pH Balance – Alkalize for Health

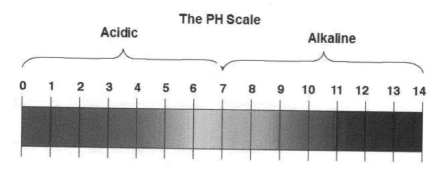

Getting your body into a more alkaline state is one of the most important and sixth step towards your Better Body. The body is very electromagnetic in nature with each cell being positive on the inside and negative on the outside of the cell. That is so the cells repel and don't stick to each other so they can move smoothly and effortlessly through the blood vessels. When the body is too acidic, the cells don't flow through vessels as well. The more alkalized your blood, the more oxygen available for your cells. The more oxygenated you are, the more energized you are. The more healthy foods and live foods you eat, the more minerals you have available. The more minerals you have, the more alive you become. The faster your cells work, the faster they recover. The quicker you detoxify. The longer you live!!

Today, many Americans have diets and lifestyles that have become extremely acidic. The foods we eat on a regular basis are very acid-forming, such as meats, pasteurized dairy products, Trans fats, refined prepackaged foods, coffee, soda, alcohol, tea, and carbonated drinks. Lifestyle habits such as lack of exercise, high stress, overloaded schedules, lack of sleep, stimulating electronic usage and taking pharmaceutical drugs all contribute to high forms of acidosis. Anxiety and living under pressure is also acid forming. Pollutions, household cleaning chemicals, and the natural aging process are all factors that lead to an acid build up in our bodies.

Benefits of an Alkaline Body System

The potential of hydrogen, or pH, ranges from 0, extremely acidic, to 14, extremely alkaline. A pH of 5 for example is 10 times as acidic as a pH of 6. The more alkaline we are, the easier it is for our blood to move throughout our bodies. Injuries, which need blood to repair, are more likely to heal faster and more completely when the surrounding tissues and blood are alkaline. In an acidic body, aging is accelerated causing our blood vessels to thicken, wrinkle and dry up.

The more acidic your cells, the harder it is for them to receive essential nutrients and oxygen, causing you to be less efficient and lethargic in our everyday functions. On the other hand, when acid waste is removed from your body, aging is slowed and you function at a higher level with greater ease.

The bottom line is that no injury or illness can repair as quickly or heal as completely without balancing pH and flushing excess acid waste from the body. If you are too acidic, you are unhealthy and will heal much more slowly, if at all.

How Does Your Body Deal With Acid

The primary organs that help our body maintain proper pH balance are the lungs and the kidneys. They both are on a constant look out to help buffer the blood or body fluids to maintain the tight range it must stay in. When the body is dehydrated or consuming a lot of toxic food or beverages, it puts more strain on the kidneys. Additionally, when you are stressed or tense, it causes more strain on your lungs. So maintaining a clean healthy lifestyle will allow your body to stay more alkalized.

There are many small things you can do to move towards an alkaline lifestyle. People often think they have to change everything and eat completely different to make a difference in their acid loads. Many times our body responds wonderfully to small simple baby steps.

To maintain optimum health or restore your health status there are a few basic rules you must follow. Remember it is all about consistency. You may have not developed a condition over night; therefore, you must realize it takes time for the body to reprogram itself and the cells. Rest assured, if you follow the basic rules, have a good attitude, and stay consistent, inevitably the body will change for the better.

Exercises, natural therapies, certain types of baths, certain foods, special minerals and supplements and certain breathing styles will all contribute to alkalizing your body. This is great, because many times you don't have to check into a treatment center, fly across the world, or spend thousands of dollars to make a massive change in your body's health.

The best way to balance your biochemistry is to eat and drink more alkaline foods and make wise lifestyle choices. Take high quality mineral formulations to buffer the pH. I recommend a company called YOLI. They have a product called ALKALETE. It is designed to buffer body acid. The product contains minerals which help to bring the body pH back towards the alkaline side of the pH scale. Patients notice almost immediate improvement after alkalizing their body. Feeding your body minerals brings more oxygen to the cells of the body, leaving you feeling more energized and healing your injuries quicker.

Alkalizing your body with exercise has a great effect on the kidneys, liver, lungs, and lymphatic system. The more you elevate your heart rate and breathing rate the more oxygenated your blood. You will move your lymph fluids through the lymphatic vessels, leaving your body cleaner and more purified.

Some other simple low cost ways to improve your health and alkalize is yoga. Yoga offers gentle stretching, increases flexibility, strength, and allows you to focus on breathing. Biking or hiking is another great way to de-stress and alkalize your body. Anytime you can connect with the outdoors your body pH and health will improve.

Virtually all food contains acids. Far fewer foods contain alkalis. The recommended 80/20 ratio of alkaline to acid foods has been reversed by the Standard Western Diet to more like 90% acidic food and 10% alkaline.

Salt and Soda baths work great too. A few times a week, soak in a hot tub of water with 1 ½ cups of Epsom salts and ¾-1 cup of baking soda. I also add a few drops of lavender oil and light a candle and put some soft relaxing music on. While you are in the tub soaking, do 5 deep diaphragm breaths and clear your mind. De-stressing will always alkalize your chemistry.

I recommend to try and exercise at least three to five times per week for body alkalization. Deep diaphragm breathing allows more oxygen into your body which alkalizes your body chemistry.

Most of us already know that exercise has so many positive health benefits. This is why you must start now, even if it is small baby steps with only 10 minutes a day working up to 20 minutes a day after a few weeks. Just start somewhere.

Make your exercise goal realistic to start with. Whatever is comfortable and attainable. I don't want it to be too much to start with and then you give up, because it was too much to keep up with.

Exercise increases your metabolism, reduces stress, builds bone mass, increases oxygen in your body, strengthens your heart muscles, releases "feel good" hormones, allows for flexibility and strength. It also improves self-confidence, relaxes your mind, and improves your sex drive.

When you exercise you sweat out your acid loads. If you sweat while exercising, you are releasing acid from stored tissues. But be careful not to over exercise. People, who do overdo it, pay the price and actually become more acidic. Too much exercise will produce too much lactic acid and cause your body to hurt and have slower recovery time.

A great way to start is 30-40 minutes three to five days a week. It is best to find time in the morning to work out, as it brings you more energy for the day. Additionally, it clears your mind and gets you mentally focused for

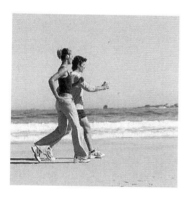

your day ahead. As you do deeper breathing with your exercise you will be oxygenating and alkalizing your body. As a result you will be detoxing your body more efficiently.

Walking is one of the best, simplest ways to oxygenate your body. A good brisk walk is best. This should not be a stroll, it should be at a pace where you are moving your arms, your legs, and focusing on deep breathing to bring oxygen throughout your system. When you breathe more deeply, you release carbon dioxide, which will decrease the acid loads in your body.

As a natural holistic chiropractic physician, I have seen firsthand how natural healing therapies work to improve health. I teach my clients how to do deep breathing. You would be amazed at how many people don't know how to take a slow deep belly breath. We call this diaphragm breathing. It is extremely successful in alkalizing the body. Deep breathing also helps with stress, pain management, lung problems, digestion problems, reducing blood pressure, and helps right before going to bed at night for a better deeper sleep.

Along with deep breathing, chiropractic, acupuncture, detoxing, supplements, teaching people about gratitude journaling, and stretching all work to reduce acid in the body.

When you turn the body's own natural self-healing mechanisms into full gear, expect miracles with holistic health and healing and find your new better body.

Daily Alkalizers

Alkalete tablets (2-4 daily). Warm water with lemon. Dry skin brush in the shower. Deep breathing daily. Daily Green salads. Yoga stretching daily. Gratitude journal. Exercise 3-5 times per week. Salt and soda baths 2-3 times per week. Get plenty of good solid sleep. Drink lots of pure fresh water. Eat extra green vegetables daily. Follow a Mediterranean type diet, high in healthy fats, nuts, seeds, vegetables, and fish.

Note: Minimize corn, carrots, potatoes, and starches. Keep red meats to a minimum.

What Our Bodies Need to be Alkaline?

With diets full of fast food, coffee, and colas, most of us are deficient in essential minerals. This deficiency contributes to the buildup of acid in our bodies. Eating fruits and vegetables is the best way to obtain a large amount and variety of alkaline minerals on a daily basis. We all have a desire to be healthy and this responsibility should include: rest, emotional balance, clean water, nutrition through proper diet, adequate sleep, regular exercise and an alkaline diet. Thomas Edison was credited with saying: "the doctor of the future will give no medicine, but will interest his patients in the care of the human frame, in diet and in the cause and prevention of disease."

If you always feel sick and tired, try to drink and eat alkaline, and exercise using a highly alkaline exercise routine. (incorporate deep breathing and no overly strenuous type workouts). By now you know that our health depends upon the balance of our inner body system and in specific our Acid/Alkaline balance. If you haven't known this until now, chances are you may already be acidic. You may also feel the symptoms of acidity like always feeling ill and fatigued, chronic headaches, aches and pains in your joints and muscles, etc. These are just some of the minor symptoms of metabolic acidosis.

Unhealthy foods such as sugar, fried foods, hydrogenated fats, foods containing too many chemicals, and foods that are too acidic, and ruin our body chemistry. There are chemical changes that occur within the relationship between minerals. When one mineral gets off balance, it can affect the others, leading into a cascade of problems.

Alkalize to Reduce Inflammation

People know when they are inflamed because they hurt. At the core of all inflammation there is an over accumulation of lactic acid or some sort of acid load. People will feel sore, tight; have pain, and possibly swelling. Many athletes or people who are highly stressed have some sort of inflammatory process taking place. Alkalizing your body will reduce the acid load and allow for a quicker recovery time, reduce the inflammation, and allow more oxygen to be readily available for the cells to repair quicker. Leaving you to feel your best. Many of today's poor lifestyle choices cause chronic inflammation include a poor diet, dehydration, stress, and sedentary living. Diet is a major key for causing or preventing inflammation. Taking the right minerals or herbs will also reduce your inflammation.

> *When pH in the brain cells is off center, appropriate chemicals are not produced and the cells can't communicate properly. This can result in insomnia, anxiety, depression, neuroses, psychoses and memory loss.*

Alkalize to Build Strong Bones

If you compare a brick wall without mortar to a brick wall with mortar to determine overall strength it's quite obvious that a brick wall's strength is dependent on the mortar. When you use this analogy for bone strength and think of the bricks as calcium and the mortar as the other 17 nutrients crucial to building strong bones it becomes very clear that simply adding more calcium (bricks) may make the wall higher, but not stronger. To build strong bones for life we need more than just brick. We also need mortar, and lots of it. If our bones were just sticks of calcium they would break as easy as chalk, but of course they're not. Bones are living cells called osteoblasts that are immobilized in a lattice work of collagen whose spaces are filled by crystals of hardened minerals, including calcium.

How Do Certain Foods Make the Blood Acidic?

Protein is the primary item that makes the blood acidic. A high – protein diet reduces the blood pH to the lower normal range, forcing the body to take steps to raise the blood's pH by extracting calcium compounds out of bone. The unique concept that YOLI has put together, is a higher protein, low carbohydrate type diet, but to counteract the acid loads, you take the pH buffering minerals to raise the mineral content in the body, preventing your body from stealing minerals from your bones to neutralize the high acid loads. It is brilliant. Now you can consume high protein, which builds and tones muscles. Eat lower carbohydrate foods to avoid increase of blood sugars or insulin levels. Finally, you take the Alkalete to buffer the pH from the higher protein diet, leaving no negative effects on the body. Brilliant!!

The Alkalizing Protocol

- **Step 1,** pH Alkalizers, take 2-4 Alkalete each morning, and pure Water(add lemon for detoxification)
- **Step 2**, eat alkaline foods throughout the day
- **Step 3**, Deep breathing daily, Yoga stretching, exercises.
- **Step 4:** Take 2-4 Alkalete tablets before bed. Additionally, Take PURE, probiotic formula.

A body that is alkalized is a healthy body. It is hard for the body to feel lousy when it is full of minerals, oxygen, has healthy greens, low stress, and proper hydration taking place. The body is happy and cooperates with you when you treat it correctly. You will live a long life when you are alkalized.

Chapter 10

Chiropractic, Acupuncture & Exercise

As a chiropractor, I know full well the importance of keeping your physical body, spine, and foundation strong and in proper alignment. You will not have ultimate health, longevity or your BETTER BODY unless you are structurally sound. Just as you would never buy a home with an unsteady or weak foundation, you cannot get the full potential out of your body and life with a weak foundation. The seventh step to your better body deals with how your physical health, foundation, and structure are important in your long term goal for health and wellness.

Back pain may be the most common reason patients seek the expertise of a chiropractor, but chiropractic techniques accomplish far more. They help patients with acute or chronic issues, including headaches, neck pain, sciatica and improper function of the nervous system that may result from car accidents, sports injuries, heredity and other causes.

Because chiropractic healthcare is holistic care, patients look to chiropractors for general wellness, too. In fact, preventive healthcare is among the fastest growing areas of chiropractic care.

According to the fountainhead of chiropractic, Palmer College of Chiropractic, chiropractic is the method of natural healing most chosen by those seeking complementary/alternative health care for acute and chronic conditions.

While you may first visit a chiropractor to relieve pain in the lower back or to treat sciatica, neck pain, whiplash or headache, you will find that a chiropractor views you as a whole person and not the sum of your parts. A chiropractor will work in partnership with you to ensure your optimal health and wellness.

Triggers Your Body's Ability to Heal

Chiropractors recognize that many factors affect your health, including exercise, nutrition, sleep, environment and heredity. Chiropractic focuses on maintaining your health naturally to help your body resist disease, rather than simply treating the symptoms of disease.

Involves No Drugs or Surgery

A broad range of techniques are used to locate, analyze and gently correct vertebral misalignments (subluxations) in the spine. Chiropractors may use manual adjustment, electrical muscular stimulation, ultrasound or massage. But they never use pharmaceutical drugs or invasive surgery. Chiropractic is a natural method of healing that stimulates the body's communication system to work more effectively to initiate, control and coordinate the various functions of the cells, organs and systems of the body. You probably may have experienced an ache or pain at some point in your life.

Others of you may have more serious health conditions. Either way, you are looking for relief. To achieve your BETTER BODY you must understand the basics on the foundation for health. The foundation starts with your physical body. You must remove interferences within the spinal, muscular, connective tissue of the body.

There are several approaches to <u>rebuilding a strong foundation</u>. Just as one would never build a house on an uneven foundation, the same is true for your physical health. You or your chiropractor must first evaluate your body for where the interferences are coming from. Once your body reveals the weak areas leading to the dysfunction, you can begin the rebuilding process.

The most important system to clear from any interference is the Central Nervous System. This is literally the "wiring system" of your body. It is crucial for the main system to be turned back on for the healing process to even begin.

There are <u>three basic causes</u> that may produce interferences in the nervous system. They are: Physical trauma, emotional stressors, and toxins that enter your body system. Eighty percent of all conditions will improve when the structure of the body is properly re-established to allow a flow of healing energy to move throughout the body. I want to educate you on the importance of your structural foundation. This is your temple and you must try your best to restore its condition. Healing the body safely and naturally without drugs or surgery is my main focus.

The Modes to Healing Physical Ailments

- ➤ **Adjustments**: use of hands or instrument to realign the spinal column to allow spinal nerves to function normal. Releases muscle tension along spine.
- ➤ **Percussion**: Soft tissue and connective tissue correction instrument.
- ➤ **Stretching**: utilizing active or passive stretches to enable proper movement in the body, connective tissues, and muscles.
- ➤ **Cold- Low Level Laser**: frequency generated laser beams cause a healing effect on the tissues of the body. Passive technique. Draws energy to help the body heal quicker. Helps to restore range of motion.
- ➤ **Pulsed –Electro Magnetic therapy**: Sending pulsed magnetic healing to certain parts of the body to remove pain and restore energy to the cells.

- ➢ **Visceral Manipulation:** Working with the organs to relieve pressure and allow normal function.
- ➢ **Acupuncture:** Used for thousands of years. Utilizing needles or electrical stimulating to certain "energetic" pathways to restore the inner energy flow of the body known as "chi". Once chi flows, dysfunction starts to improve.
- ➢ **Ultrasound:** deep penetrating ultrasonic heat waves to break up scar tissue, tension, and knots in the body.
- ➢ **Electric stimulation:** small pads placed on skin sending electrical stimulus to the muscles to relax and relieve pain.

Once your chiropractor has decided which mode or combination of techniques to incorporate you most likely will feel a difference within the first few visits. Depending on the duration of the problem it may take a few weeks to make a change in your physical foundation. Also, sometimes you may feel worse before you feel better. This is because your joints, muscles, and bones may have been so misaligned that you are changing the pattern of the body. Nevertheless, by re-establishing a strong nervous system the entire body will benefit and health returns.

There Are Three Phases of Care:

1. **Relief care:**
   works on removing muscle tension, pain or spasms. Also works on initial subluxation, vertebral misalignment putting pressure or inflammation on surrounding nerves.

2. **Corrective care:**
   Once initial relief has been established, this is the phase where we reeducate your body, the patterns, and continue providing supportive adjustments or therapy to avoid falling back into pain or symptomology.

3. **Maintenance or Wellness care:**
   Completely preventative in nature for your health. We believe this should be the goal of most people. Problems will most likely not return. If they should arise again, your body will respond with speed because your body has been conditioned for real health through regular chiropractic care.

Your visits may be frequent during the relief care phase. You are re-establishing a new structural pattern. Each visit will build on the ones before, so keeping your appointments will bring best results. Your body will need to be re-educated on the "new" positions your chiropractor is trying to put in place. This takes time. Be patient through this process and realize the effort you put into your healing will be what you get out of your healing process.

I tell my patients, my reputation and your results are of the upmost importance to me. I would like to ask you to respect our natural healing avenues of chiropractic, acupuncture, and the other healing modalities. If you are only wanting to "try" something one time; please realize you will most likely not get the results you are looking for in one single treatment. Wellness care takes time and many changes in our habits and daily choices.

To achieve permanent and lasting results, a strong foundation must be built. This is done by addressing the whole person, with structural care being one of the major steps in your Better Body. The other avenues to address are: nutritional, emotional, detoxing, lifestyle changes, balancing body pH, balancing hormones, balancing blood sugars.

Exercise

Most of us are non-exercisers. Even though we believe in exercise—90 percent of Americans rate exercise as essential to good health. We just don't do it—only 20 percent of Americans actually exercise. No matter how old you are or what shape you're in, it's never too late to get moving to help your body last longer and be stronger.

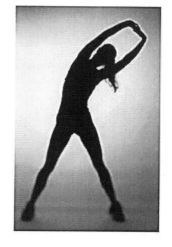

Along with watching what you eat, exercising is about the best thing you can do for yourself. But if you just exercise, without watching what you eat, you're only doing yourself about half as much good. For one thing, exercise puts certain demands on your body that you have to compensate for.

One of them is calories. The more you exercise whether it is a four-mile run, an hour-long aerobics class, or a regular game of racquetball, the more calories your body's going to burn.

Why Exercise?

Some benefits of a regular exercise program are obvious: improved appearance, weight control, and overall better health. But others are more hidden – for example, physical exercise throughout life can actually slow the loss of calcium from the body and help prevent bond degeneration, or osteoporosis, in old age. Regular exercise can not only extend your life – middle-aged people with desk jobs who don't exercise are twice as susceptible to heart attacks as those who do – but can also improve the quality of your life.

For your exercise routine to be effective, you need to perform it at least three times a week, a minimum of 20 continuous minutes each session, during which you maintain your heartbeat (pulse) between 70 and 85 percent of its maximum capability. To help you stick to your routine, choose exercises that you enjoy and if you can exercise with a friend.

Have you ever heard the expression "use it or lose it"? It's true! If you don't use your body, you will surely lose it. Your muscles will become flabby and weak. Your heart and lungs won't function efficiently. And your joints will be stiff and easily injured. Inactivity is as much of a health risk as smoking!

Helps Prevent Diseases

Our bodies were meant to move -- they actually crave exercise. Regular exercise is necessary for physical fitness and good health. It reduces the risk of heart disease, cancer, high blood pressure, diabetes and other diseases. It can improve your appearance and delay the aging process.

Improves Stamina

When you exercise, your body uses energy to keep going. Aerobic exercise involves continuous and rhythmic physical motion, such as walking and bicycling. It improves your stamina by training your body to become more efficient and use less energy for the same amount of work. As your conditioning level improves, your heart rate and breathing rate return to resting levels much sooner from strenuous activity.

Strengthens and Tones

Exercising with weights and other forms of resistance training develops your muscles, bones and ligaments for increased strength and endurance. Your posture can be improved, and your muscles become more firm and toned. You not only feel better, but you look better, too!

Enhances Flexibility

Stretching exercises are also important for good posture. They keep your body limber so that you can bend, reach and twist. Improving your flexibility through exercise reduces the chance of injury and improves balance and coordination. If you have stiff, tense areas, such as the upper back or neck, performing specific stretches can help "loosen" those muscles, helping you feel more relaxed.

Controls Weight

Exercise is also a key to weight control because it burns calories. If you burn off more calories than you take in, you lose weight. It's as simple as that.

Improves Quality of Life

Once you begin to exercise regularly, you will discover many more reasons why exercise is so important to improving the quality of your life. Exercise reduces stress, lifts moods, and helps you sleep better. It can keep you looking and feeling younger throughout your entire life.

Exercise does wonderful things for your body. It releases endorphins, which are "feel-good" neurotransmitters, or brain chemicals, which literally make you feel better. That's why some depression can be treated with consistent exercise

Studies show that four hours of exercise a week reduces a woman's risk of breast cancer by 60 percent! That alone makes it worth the effort for any woman. In fact, exercise has been shown to reduce the risk of colon cancer, pancreatic cancer, and prostate cancer too. Exercise can also prevent, control, and even reverse adult-onset diabetes (because it reduces fat and allows insulin to start working again). Given the high incidence of diabetes these days, which make exercise worth the effort for anyone. I can't think of one ailment that exercise wouldn't hugely benefit.

Acupuncture

Acupuncture, simply stated, is a health science which is used to successfully treat both pain and dysfunction in the body. Acupuncture has its roots deeply planted in China. In fact, authorities agree the science is between 5,000 and 7,000 years old. Acupuncture is the utilization of needles placed in the skin at various locations to relieve pain or affect a body part. Early Chinese physicians discovered there is an energy network traversing just below the surface of the skin which communicates from the exterior to the internal organs and structures at over 1,000 "Acupoints" on the body. This energy works in harmony with the body's circulatory, nervous, muscular, digestive, genitourinary and all other systems of the body. When this vital energy becomes blocked or weakened, an effect in a body system or anatomic location becomes evident. Stimulation of one or a combination of key "Acupoints" on the body may restore harmony to the affected area.

Historians have stated, "More people have benefited from Acupuncture over the course of fifty centuries than the combined total of all other healing sciences, both ancient and modern." Acupuncture is a principle, not a technique. Many practitioners use electronic stimulation, laser beam or pressure massage to treat an Acupoint. The principle of Acupuncture does not change, only the technique.

The human body's energy flow courses over twelve meridians or channels that are normally well balanced. If a disruption of energy flow exists, it can alter the entire system, producing pain or symptoms in the body. This is acupuncture's goal-to restore normalcy to the body's energy balance by utilizing a combination of Acupoints located on the twelve meridians. This is accomplished by a variety of means, the needle is just one. Four acupuncture needles can easily be inserted into the hollow tube of a hypodermic needle. Because of the extreme slenderness of the needle, most people compare the sensations "less than a mosquito bite." Acupuncturists are employing electronic and laser stimulation to the Acupoint with equal effectiveness as the needle. Both of these procedures are painless and are quickly becoming standard worldwide.

Some patients notice an immediate improvement after the first treatment, whereas others may not notice any effect until the seventh or eighth visit. It has been shown that a certain percentage of patients receive maximum benefit up to three months following a course of therapy. The usual number of treatments is between eight and sixteen. The usual frequency is between two and four times a week.

What Conditions are Accepted

Acute and chronic pain relief, migraine, tension cluster and sinus headaches, trigeminal neuralgia, bladder dysfunction, bed wetting, cervical(neck) pain, and mid-back pain, low shoulder, tennis elbow, post-operative pain relief, gastric problems, asthma, allergies, skin conditions, hemorrhoids, abnormal blood pressure, fatigue, anxiety, neurologic syndrome, various eye problems, etc., etc. This is only a partial list of the numerous conditions Acupuncture has been credited with helping.

Acupuncture has gained a great deal of notoriety in recent years concerning its considerable success with addiction control. It has been shown that Acupuncture has a very positive effect in the area of both drug and alcohol addiction. One of the most noteworthy addictions Acupuncture helps is smoking. The average patient will reduce their intake by at least one half within twenty four hours of the first treatment.

So you can now see how important having your body in proper alignment and getting adequate exercise can be. All it takes are baby steps, a small change each week can yield giant dividends in the future. What step will you take today? The choice is yours.

Chapter 11

Healthy Gut – Happy Body

"All disease begins in the gut." Hippocrates said this more than 2,000 years ago, but we're only now coming to understand just how right he was. Having a healthy gut is the eighth step in obtaining your BETTER BODY.

As a holistic wellness practitioner, I believe one of the first things you must get working is the gut for health to return. You cannot expect a person to achieve ultimate health with an unhealthy digestive system. That is where they absorb their nutrients and get rid of their toxins. The gut is known to be the key to long life.

There are two things you MUST do to start healing your Temple: Start on Probiotics and Digestive Enzymes. Probiotics are capsules you take daily that help bring lots of extra good bacteria into your body. This good bacteria is like extra protection for your gut and your immune system. I think of it like the army that protects you from foreign invaders. And there are lots of foreign invaders, such as virus, bad bacteria, parasites, fungus, molds, chemicals, and more. The probiotics you take on a daily basis will help you with protecting your health, building your immune system, and most importantly protecting your entire mucus membrane path (nose, mouth, lungs, guts, rectum, and the whole "tube" from top to bottom).

Enzymes help to break down your food and all other materials in your body. Most people just don't have enough digestive enzymes due to stress, medications, or poor lifestyle. Taking enzymes and probiotics are like a miracle combination for immune function, health, allergies, and digestive function. Everyone should be on both!

My goal is to get your gut as healthy as possible by the end of you reading this book. I want you to realize you need to be digesting your foods properly, and eliminating waste daily and efficiently. I will give you a step by step process to get the entire digestive system working again.

Our gut is home to approximately 100,000,000,000,000 (100 trillion) microorganisms. That's such a big number our human brains can't really comprehend it. One trillion dollar bills laid end-to-end would stretch from the earth to the sun – and back – with a lot of miles to spare. Do that 100 times and you start to get at least a vague idea of how much 100 trillion is. (Kresser, 2012)

We've only recently begun to understand the extent of the gut flora's role in human health and disease. Among other things, the gut flora promotes normal gastrointestinal function, provides protection from infection, regulates metabolism and comprises more than 75% of our immune system.

Antibiotics are very harmful to the gut flora. Recent studies have shown that antibiotic use causes a profound and rapid loss of diversity and a shift in the composition of the gut flora. Without some intervention, the variety of healthy gut flora cannot be recovered after the use of antibiotics.

It is a real tragedy that when a person is put on antibiotics, they are not put on probiotics as well to rebuild the healthy bacteria in the gut. As you probably know, when you take antibiotics, they kill harmful bacteria, but they also kill beneficial bacteria (probiotics). After you're done with a round of antibiotics, your intestines will slowly try to come back to their former balance, but in our pasteurized, sterilized world, this is more difficult than it used to be. And besides, antibiotics don't kill everything. They hardly affect yeast, which is usually only about one percent of our intestinal microbe population. But with its bacterial competition out of the way because of the antibiotics, yeasts can flourish.

The more rounds of antibiotics we endure, the more out of balance our intestinal ecosystem can become, and this lack of microbial balance can create problems — problems that can be solved by deliberately re-introducing beneficial bacteria (probiotics) into your diet.

There are several other things that contribute to an imbalance in our bacteria. Most important (besides antibiotics) is what we eat. Sugar selectively feeds harmful bacteria. Fiber selectively feeds beneficial bacteria. So as our diet has changed, the kinds of bacteria living in our guts have changed too. We also aren't exposed to as many bacteria as we once were because of chlorine in our drinking water, antibacterial soaps and hand gels, etc. This means if you want to have a healthy micro flora, you're going to have to take deliberate steps to make it happen.

It is also known that if infants aren't breast-fed and are born to mothers with bad gut flora are more likely to develop unhealthy gut bacteria, and that these early differences in gut flora may predict overweight, diabetes, eczema/psoriasis, depression and other health problems in the future.

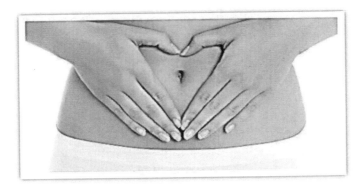

The gut barrier is the gatekeeper that decides what gets in and what stays out. The immune system goes on high alert with this and wants to attack the large proteins. There is a direct correlation of the digestive health and overall immune function.

There is no health without a healthy gut. The gut has three functions crucial to your health: (1) it breaks food down to nutrients; (2) it absorbs those nutrients into the blood through the intestinal walls, and (3) prevents foreign and toxic molecules from entering the bloodstream. Add to it that a healthy intestine has a major role in detoxification by neutralizing or breaking down toxins ingested with food and it becomes clear that any gut malfunction will adversely affect health.

You can eat the best foods, keep your exposure to toxins low and keep the brightest, most positive attitude, but if your digestion, nutrient absorption and gut-detoxification are not functioning properly, your health will deteriorate.

How wide-spread are various forms of malfunctioning, unhealthy gut? While no exact numbers are known, the estimate is that well over 100 million Americans live with impaired digestion.

It is no wonder, with low-fiber diets based on meat and processed foods, causing many issues with our digestive tracts and our whole bodies. This can, and regularly does cause or contribute to symptoms of indigestion, as well as many other symptoms directly or indirectly associated with it.

Many are not aware of having food sensitivities and allergies, or inflamed intestines. Often times, not because of the absence of symptoms, but because:

    A. food sensitivities most often don't show at the time of food consumption, and

    B. common symptoms of not feeling well are seldom seen as related to gut condition.

About one in every four Americans has so called "irritable bowel". This is not a diagnosis, but merely a descriptive label covering variety of digestive disturbances with their own sub-labels, from IBS (Irritable Bowel Syndrome) and colitis, to Crohn's disease.

Food Sensitivities

What would cause unhealthy gut? One possible reason is food sensitivities and allergies. They can be result of genetic deficiency, preventing synthesis of enzymes needed for proper digestion of certain food components, immune system malfunction, reaction to chemical additives, and other factors.

Poorly digested food molecules feed harmful bacteria, irritating intestines and causing immune response. It leads into chronic inflammation of the intestinal lining and compromised digestion, usually accompanied with over-growth of harmful, toxic bacteria and/or fungi.

> *Your colon is one of the primary channels of elimination of toxic waste in your body. If your colon is functioning properly you should have a bowel movement after every primary meal.*

This may and may not cause significant abdominal discomfort, or pain (keep in mind that the body often quickly adapts to unfavorable conditions, but there is usually a price to pay down the road). However, it always hampers digestion and absorption of nutrients, as inflammation and toxicity of the intestines worsen. Carrier proteins transporting nutrients across the membrane into the blood are damaged, and so is the nutrient-absorbing intestinal lining, whose functional area can be reduced to a small fraction of its normal size.

Your nutritional status deteriorates, and it is only question of time when the integrity of intestinal membrane is compromised.

What happens next is the condition called leaky gut syndrome, where undigested food proteins begin to penetrate the inflamed intestinal membrane, get into the bloodstream, and provoke formation of new antibodies by the immune system. These new, abnormal (since formed against large food molecules that shouldn't be present in the blood, and may have immune markers similar to our tissue molecules) antibodies sometimes mistakenly attack body organs and tissues, causing mysterious symptoms, multiple food sensitivities and food allergies, arthritic symptoms, asthma symptoms, or serious auto-immune diseases like rheumatoid arthritis, lupus, myocarditis, multiple sclerosis or Lou Gehrig's disease.

It is not only undigested protein molecules that leak through the inflamed intestinal lining. Intestinal toxins also penetrate into the blood. They can affect any organ or tissue in the body, causing random body aches (fibromyalgia), brain fog, chronic fatigue, depression, chemical sensitivities due to the overwhelmed detox system, and so on.

Leaky gut also allows potentially harmful microorganisms to migrate from the intestine to any part of the body, further compromising its integrity.

Specific ailments caused by leaky gut vary widely from one individual to another, depending on the complex interaction of individual strengths and weaknesses. There are specific formulas for Leaky Gut.

Your Steps Towards a Healthy Gut and a Better Body

One of the first steps in healing the lining of your intestinal tract is identifying possible food allergies. Many times the whole cascade starts with the gut. Food allergies may be occurring without you even knowing. These are called functional food allergies. What this means is you can eat certain foods which can cause many of your symptoms, such as headaches, dizziness, fatigue, or even weight gain. These foods will not cause you to die or have major problems, but always keeps the "fire" going.

I recommend cleaning up your diet. This means going back to the nutrition chapter and eating the foods recommended and avoiding the sugary, fried, or processed unhealthy foods. Many times this will do the trick along with a few other recommendations. If this doesn't work, I recommend the ELIMINATION DIET. This means you will eliminate certain foods to see if symptoms improve.

You will want to avoid a certain food for several weeks to try to shut off the inflammatory response. Once you eliminate a certain food group, such as dairy or gluten, and symptoms improve, stay off that particular food group for possibly several months. Each case is different and many times there is an underlying cause that has started the food allergies, such as adrenal fatigue or high stress. If the underlying causes are being eliminated, many times food allergies can be reversed, meaning they are only temporary. There are other times, where you may have to stay away from a certain food group for years or a lifetime. You may be able to eat the foods, but you will notice each time you do eat the "offending food", you will get headaches, fatigue, skin rashes, or any other symptom.

I typically recommend the elimination diet with dairy, wheat, corn, soy, or even food additives (such as avoiding everything with aspartame or MSG).

Once you have started cleaning up your diet, eliminating certain foods, now it is time to start with supplements, stress management, and other holistic healing options.

Recommendations

I put people on Digestive plant based enzymes with each meal. I recommend you take 1-2 with each meal and slightly before you eat. Along with enzymes I recommend taking Probiotics at bedtime. This is due to the fact the live bacteria can have a chance to work on re-establishing healthy digestive flora while you sleeping.

Finally, L-Glutamine, slippery elm, aloe vera, Jerusalem artichoke are also great remedies to take daily to promote digestive healing. Enzymes and probiotics are a must for long term digestive health. Even without digestive problems, I still recommend taking these two supplements for overall health, immunity, and energy. This is definitely part of the Better body plan.

Acupuncture works wonderful for healing digestive problems. I have witnessed hundreds of cases of digestive problems be resolved from a series of acupuncture treatments. Acupuncture restores the energetic flow within the body and opens the meridian channels, drawing extra healing energy to the gut region.

Chiropractic adjustments around the middle of the back allows for the nerve impulses to get from the brain to the digestive tract. If the spinal bones are out of alignment, it will not allow for full health to be taking place at certain organs, glands, or body parts. Chiropractic gives you a chance to receive an actual treatment to try and heal your digestive system quicker.

Emotional stress and worry will always cause more digestive disturbance, as it shuts off your parasympathetic nervous system. I recommend you do deep breathing, stress management techniques listed in this book. Additionally, a warm compress to the belly will calm down stress and help the gut region feel better. It is very soothing.

Along with the supplements, modifying the foods, doing chiropractic and acupuncture, you can try using peppermint and ginger into your daily regimen. You may use peppermint essential oil and follow instructions. Additionally, ginger has long been used for healing the gut. I recommend using fresh ginger or making a tea.

The gut is the key to your health. The gut makes many of your vitamins. I would follow the supplementation protocols and work on reducing your stress and watch your digestive health improve before your eyes. You will no longer be a prisoner to your house needing a restroom nearby. You will no longer need to be buying rolls of antacids.

Chapter 12

Inflammation – Warning System

You have all experienced inflammation at different times. When you think of pain, red hot, burning, throbbing, hurting, stabbing, or piercing you can rest assure there is an inflammatory response taking place. The ninth step to a better body deals with reducing inflammation.

What people don't realize is they can have lingering chronic inflammation causing them to never feel quite right. Low grade infections, chronic stress, poor diets, repetitive motions at work, excessive activity, sports, headaches, chronic illnesses or infections all have inflammation occurring on a cellular level.

If you stub your toe or twist your ankle, you know you are in immediate inflammation. It hurts!! It swells up. It starts to throb. The physical symptoms of swelling and pain, part of the process known as acute inflammation, are typically short lived and are a necessary part of your initial recovery.

Inflammation is Not Always From a Physical Injury

There are a number of disorders, including obesity and joint pain, which are brought on by chronic subclinical inflammation. Experts believe that chronic inflammation is now a major problem in our society, primarily due to our diet and high stress levels.

The foods that we typically eat promote both inflammation and weight gain, and the excess fat leads us on a vicious cycle, causing more inflammation, creating the mess people end up in.

People gain weight, as a result their joints hurt so then they don't exercise, which leaves their body to gain more weight, and since they hurt and are gaining weight, they tend to eat "comfort" foods, which are typically sugar or fast foods. So the cycle of inflammation continues.

Luckily, the inflammatory process can be avoided and even reversed. By making smart choices in the foods you put into your body and using carefully thought out nutrients, herbs, minerals, vitamins, water, light activity, positive thinking, you can eliminate chronic inflammation and enjoy a stronger healthier body.

Many times you may even be able to put certain auto-immune diseases into remission or start the healing process on serious diseases by putting out the fire.

What is Chronic Inflammation?

Inflammation is a cellular process used to heal destroyed or damaged tissues. It is protective in nature. Your body is trying to put out a fire to say the least. The process is designed to defend the body against harmful substances like virus, bacteria, parasites, harmful chemicals, dead tissues, foreign invaders, broken cells, sick cells, acid overload, or unhealthy food.

It's like an army, it wants to clear out the bad, and send in extra protection. It wants to surround the bad areas with extra special forces. That is where swelling comes from. That is your body laying down extra fluid to protect something that is in danger. Think of someone with arthritis, their joints hurt; so many times the joints become swollen. There is extra cellular activity going on at that location.

Inflammation is trying to promote renewal of healthy tissue. When the body becomes injured, say you cut your finger on a piece of glass, your body releases chemicals such as histamines or prostaglandins, which make the blood vessels react to increase the blood flow to the injury site. As a result, the injury site swells up, becomes hot, pressure builds, all because there has been an increase in cellular activity.

Black cherries inhibit an enzyme called xanthine oxidase, a major source of harmful free radicals. Black cherries have also been found to relieve symptoms of gout and arthritis.

Many of us are familiar with an overactive immune response and too much inflammation. It results in common conditions like allergies, rheumatoid arthritis, autoimmune disease, and asthma. This is bad inflammation, and if it is left unchecked it can become downright ugly.

What few people understand is that hidden inflammation run amok is at the root of all chronic illness we experience -- conditions like heart disease, obesity, diabetes, dementia, depression, cancer, and even autism.

The real concern is not our response to immediate injury, infection, or insult. It is the chronic, smoldering inflammation that slowly destroys our organs and our ability to function optimally and leads to rapid aging.

Common treatments such as anti-inflammatory drugs (ibuprofen or aspirin) and steroids like prednisone -- though often useful for acute problems -- interfere with the body's own immune response and can lead to serious and deadly side effects.

In fact, as many people die from taking anti-inflammatory drugs like ibuprofen every year as die from asthma or leukemia. Stopping these drugs would be equivalent to finding the cure for asthma or leukemia -- that's a bold statement, but the data is there to back it up.

How to Locate the Causes of Hidden Inflammation

So if inflammation and immune imbalances are at the root of most of modern disease, how do we find the causes and get the body back in balance?

First, we need to identify the triggers and causes of inflammation. Then we need to help reset the body's natural immune balance by providing the right conditions for it to thrive.

We need to find those inflammatory factors unique to each person and to see how various lifestyle, environmental, or infectious factors spin the immune system out of control, leading to a host of chronic illnesses.

Many autoimmune diseases have an underlying inflammatory response taking place. To help with auto-immune diseases such as Rheumatoid arthritis, diabetes, Alzheimer's, heart disease, Ulcerative colitis we must try to reduce overall inflammation coming from external sources. This will help reduce the symptoms of the autoimmune disorders and give them a fighting chance to go into remission.

External Sources that Cause Inflammation

• Poor diet--mostly sugar, refined flours, processed foods, and inflammatory fats such as trans and saturated fats

• Lack of exercise

• Stress

• Hidden or chronic infections with viruses, bacteria, yeasts, or parasites

• Hidden allergens from food or the environment

• Toxins such as mercury and pesticides

• Mold toxins and allergens

12 Steps to Living an Anti-inflammatory Life

So once you have figured out the causes of inflammation in your life, gotten rid of them, the next step is to keep living an anti-inflammatory lifestyle. But how do you do that?

Here is what I recommend. It's a disarmingly simple but extraordinarily effective way to achieve your BETTER BODY.

1. Whole Foods - Eat a whole foods, high-fiber, plant-based diet, which is inherently anti-inflammatory. That means choosing unprocessed, unrefined, whole, fresh, real foods, not those full of sugar and trans fats and low in powerful anti-inflammatory plant chemicals called phytonutrients.
2. Healthy Fats - Give yourself an oil change by eating healthy monounsaturated fats in olive oil, nuts and avocadoes, and getting more omega-3 fats from small fish like sardines, herring, sable, and wild salmon.
3. Regular Exercise - Mounting evidence tells us that regular exercise reduces inflammation. It also improves immune function, strengthens your cardiovascular systems, corrects and prevents insulin resistance, and is key for improving your mood and erasing the effects of stress. In fact, regular exercise is one among a small handful of lifestyle changes that correlates with improved health in virtually ALL of the scientific literature. So get moving already!
4. Relax - Learn how to engage your vagus nerve by actively relaxing. This powerful nerve relaxes your whole body and lowers inflammation when you practice yoga or meditation, breathe deeply, or even take a hot bath.
5. Avoid Allergens - If you have food allergies, find out what you're allergic to and stop eating those foods—gluten, dairy and nightshade(tomatoes, potatoes and peppers) are common culprits.
6. Heal Your Gut - Take probiotics to help your digestion and improve the balance of healthy bacteria in your gut, which reduces inflammation.
7. Supplement - Take a multivitamin/multi-mineral supplement, fish oil, and vitamin D, all of which help reduce inflammation.

8. Herbal Remedies- Ginger, curcumin, ashwaganda, rhodiolia, boswellia, bromelain are a few natural herbals which are known to reduce inflammation and pain.

9. Balance your pH – Reduce acidity in your body. Acid overload in the body causes a wide range of inflammatory problems. Use Alkalete by YOLI to help cut down the acid load.

10. Gargle with Salt Water - Salt water draws moisture out of any bacteria that have set up shop there, and it draws moisture out of your own swollen tissues, relieving inflammation. It changes the pH of your throat to promote healing, and a salty environment prevents bacteria from growing

11. Reduce or Eliminate all Dairy products – this is beneficial when dealing with lung congestion, bronchitis, sinus infections and any other illness that increases mucus.

12. Reduce Sugar and Carbohydrate Intake – these reduce immune function and fuel inflammation. You will never shut down the inflammation process if you continue to eat or drink sugar.

Taking this comprehensive approach to inflammation and balancing your immune system addresses one of the most important core systems of the body.

I cannot stress this enough, at the bottom of all health problems there is an inflammatory process taking place. You must learn to keep inflammation reduce or eliminate it all together. You don't have to have swelling or pain to have inflammation. It can be on a cellular level. You will need to take precaution to keep inflammation at bay, keep your health optimal and preventing disease.

Chapter 13

Sleep – Get Re-energized

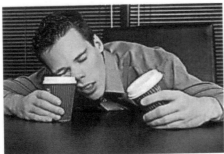

In this country, it is normal for us to work at least 10 hours a day, try to exercise a few hours a week and try to get by on 5-6 hours of sleep a night. We use alarm clocks, coffee, chocolate, soda, energy drinks and many other tricks to help us "push through" the fatigue and get on with our day. Does this sound like you? Getting adequate sleep to re-energize and revitalize is the tenth step in your journey to your BETTER BODY.

What you don't know is how exceedingly important sleep is and how not getting enough sleep can cause us to gain weight. **Just one or two nights of missed or inadequate sleep are enough to make you as insulin resistant as a Type II diabetic!** While adequate diet and exercise can help, your physiology will never be normal without enough sleep. At the end of the day, neglected sleep or poor sleep quality is a significant stressor to your body. It compromises your immune system, reduces your memory and makes you gain weight.

When you sleep, your brain goes through the previous day's experiences, primes your memory, and triggers the release of hormones regulating energy, mood, and mental acuity. To complete its work, the brain needs 7 to 8 hours of sleep. When it gets less, your concentration, creativity, mood regulation, and productivity all take a hit.

Getting More From the Sleep You Get

Given the demands the majority of people today -- working in a 24/7, always-on environment is a big one -- a full night's sleep is sometimes an impossible dream. Fortunately, there are ways to get more out of the time you do manage to spend in sleep:

- **Avoid caffeine.** Cut out caffeinated coffee, tea, and soda ideally 10 hours before bedtime -- and chocolate, too. When you sleep, make it a commitment.

- **Darken the room completely.** Your brain creates a hormone called melatonin that senses when it's dark out and primes you for sleep. If you try to sleep amid too much light, your brain may decide you're not ready for bedtime after all. So turns off the TV, shut down the computer, turn the clock to the wall, and close the blinds tightly. Use an eye mask if you're sleeping during the daytime.

- **Sleep in a restful environment.** Make sure the room is quiet and your cell phone is out of hearing range. Sleep on a comfortable mattress

- **Exploit the power of power naps**
  Don't forget that brief day-time naps can be helpful. If at all

possible, close your office door (if you have one) and try to doze for 10 to 20 minutes.

But keep the naps short. With a longer nap, you're likely to wake up while in deep sleep and feel worse than before. It can take up to 30 minutes to feel fully alert after awakening from deep sleep.

By keeping your nap to 10-20 minutes, you should be able to achieve stage 2 in the sleep cycle and wake up energized rather than groggy. A short power nap should provide enough of a boost to keep your performance going strong the rest of the day -- and is more effective (as well as healthier) than a cup of coffee.

> *Most people require at least 7 hours of sleep per night. It is during this time that your body produces collagen and elastin; two proteins which help your skin stay smooth and look younger.*

Get to Bed on Time

Actuarial figures from insurance companies show that people who go longer than seven days on five hours or fewer of sleep a night increase their risk of death from all causes by 700 percent! That's an astronomical increase.

Studies show that the hours from 10 p.m. until 2 a.m. are the most healing, restorative hours to rest - don't miss those hours of sleep. From 10 p.m. until midnight your sleep is four times more restorative than the hours you sleep after midnight, so try especially hard not to miss those hours.

Your stomach needs good rest every night too. If you get plenty of sleep but still wake up tired, maybe you aren't letting your stomach rest when you rest. Have you ever noticed that eating a big meal right before bedtime can disturb your rest or even keep you awake at night? Don't load up your stomach before bed so that it has to keep working hard all night to digest your late-night snacks. Instead, follow the maxim "Eat like a king at breakfast, a prince at lunch, and a pauper at dinner. It will do your stomach and your sleep habits a world of good.

In 1735, Ben Franklin cited another maxim in his almanac: "Early to bed and early to rise, makes a man healthy, wealthy, and wise."

Mind Over Matters

Many of us also suffer from RMS—restless mind syndrome! You are so tired, that bed feels so good, but your brain just won't shut up. One way to quiet the mind is through affirmations, meditation or quiet prayer and reflection to God's word before you retire.

Mellow Out With Melatonin

Another factor, imbalanced melatonin production can wreak havoc on your sleep cycle. Melatonin is a hormone that enables deep, healthy sleep. Older folks tend to produce less melatonin than they need at night and more during the day when it causes drowsiness. Sleeping in total darkness can help restore a balanced melatonin production schedule. Melatonin is also available in supplemental form.

Six Reasons To Get Enough Sleep

1. **Learning and memory**: Sleep helps the brain commit new information to memory through a process called memory consolidation. In studies, people who'd slept after learning a task did better on tests later.

2. **Metabolism and weight**: Chronic sleep deprivation may cause weight gain by affecting the way our bodies process and store carbohydrates, and by altering levels of hormones that affect our appetite.

3. **Safety**: Sleep debt contributes to a greater tendency to fall asleep during the daytime. These lapses may cause falls and mistakes such as medical errors, air traffic mishaps, and road accidents.

4. **Mood**: Sleep loss may result in irritability, impatience, inability to concentrate, and moodiness. Too little sleep can also leave you too tired to do the things you like to do.

5. **Cardiovascular health**: Serious sleep disorders have been linked to hypertension, increased stress hormone levels, and irregular heartbeat.

6. **Disease**: Sleep deprivation alters immune function, including the activity of the body's killer cells. Keeping up with sleep may also help fight cancer.

Holistic Approaches to Improving Sleep

1. Chiropractic adjustments: improve the function of the entire nervous system.
2. Acupuncture: Restores inner balance of the bodies subtle energies. Allowing for a more restful deep sleep.
3. Hormonal balancing: many times low progesterone will cause insomnia. Additionally, all hormones work together for the proper deep peaceful sleep. Along with reducing hot flashes, will also help you sleep better.
4. Evaluate cortisol levels. If you have high cortisol at night you will have a hard time falling asleep. You may need certain supplements to lower cortisol at night time.
5. Evaluate neurotransmitters: the brain chemistry allows our brain to shut down and find a relaxed state. If you have a hard time shutting your brain down, you should have a urine test to evaluate your brain's neurotransmitters.
6. Low Level Laser Therapy: Frequencies can be generated to rebalance the body and mind to promote sleep and relaxation
7. 5-HTP : Tryptophan is an amino acid that helps with sleep.
8. Valerian Root
9. Passion Flower
10. Kava Kava
11. Melatonin
12. Meditation and deep breathing
13. Relaxing soft music

To ensure a good night's rest, it is best to sleep in a completely dark room. Even a small amount of light will interfere with your body's circadian rhythm and pineal gland's production of melatonin and serotonin.

A nice herbal product that I use in my practice if anyone is dealing with insomnia or sleeping issues is called DREAM. It is a product produced from a company named YOLI.

Adequate sleep is a cornerstone to good health. Taking small steps can lead to a better functioning mind and body. Turn off the TV, computer and your smart phone 30 minutes earlier to relax your mind and prepare for bed. Go to bed 10 minutes earlier every day for a week, all of a sudden you have given yourself the gift of an extra hour of sleep. You can do it!

Chapter 14

Deep Breathing, Oxygen and Sunlight

One of the common denominators to rejuvenating health is learning how to incorporate deep breathing into your daily routine. This cannot be overseen as "too simple to make a difference". Many times I do everything to a patient to help with their healing process, but when I teach them some deep breathing techniques, their healing excels. Developing deep breathing techniques to increase oxygen intake and getting adequate sunlight are the eleventh step to your BETTER BODY.

If you are like most people, you are doing the majority of your breathing as short shallow breaths. This is in part from stress and hectic lifestyles. What our body yearns for is slow deep relaxed breaths. This doesn't happen naturally; most times you have to force time in your schedule daily to make this happen. This is a key to health. Make time for deep belly breathing daily. Ten deep breaths before you go to bed each night is perfect. IN through the nose and out through the mouth.

When you hold your breath or take shallow breaths, you are not allowing oxygen to reach all parts of your body. In addition, you are accumulating carbon dioxide, which is acidic and needs to be expelled from the body through exhalation. If it builds up in the blood it reacts with water to form carbonic acid, which causes a drop in the blood's pH.

If you learn to deep breath on a regular basis, your energy will improve, your moods will improve and your body will recover and heal quicker. Research shows that breathing deeply for even 30 seconds has a substantial effect on acidic stress hormones and, when practiced over time, can have a profound healing effect on mood, energy levels, and cardiovascular and respiratory health. Research collected for the National Center for Health Statistics 2002 National Health Interview Survey illustrated that deep breathing was the fourth most common complementary and alternative medicine therapy used by respondents, with almost 12 percent having done it in the preceding months.

> *Slow, deep breathing brings air to the lowest part of your lungs and exercises your diaphragm. Deep breathing relaxes your mind and body, massages your internal organs, calms emotions and promotes restful sleep.*

Meditation

Imagine your favorite beach front destination. You can hear the waves rhythmically rolling in. You can smell the ocean air, you can hear the seagulls, and you can feel the soft white sand in between your toes. You can feel the warm sun beating down on you. Feel yourself relaxing. Feel your mood relaxing. Release the tension in your neck and shoulders. Feel it. Imagine it. Breathe and just relax. Enjoy it for a moment.

Meditation can be extremely effective in achieving an alkaline body due to reduced stress. Chemicals such as cortisol, adrenaline, and others perform an important function, they are designed to help us to "flight or fight". Stress many times causes people to turn towards acidic habits, such as smoking, drinking, sugary foods, fast foods, inactivity, depressing outlooks, and self-medications.

Meditation can be a useful tool to reduce stress and open up the diaphragm. Additionally, it can help open up the acupuncture meridian channels, allowing the body to relax and return towards a more optimal state of health. Meditation has been around for thousands of years and beyond. It has been thought to be rooted in religious and spiritual traditions, meditation now has become a widespread practice for coping, relaxing, and promoting overall wellness. It can be conducted as a stand-alone technique or integrated into practices such as yoga, tai chi, deep-breathing exercises, or qigong.

Massage Therapy

This technique has been shown to be effective in reducing sore muscles and stiffness. It is also great for stress reduction, as when someone gently massages your muscles, it releases endorphins, and certain chemicals that leave you feeling good. Additionally, massage reduces the stress hormones that are circulating through your body.

Oxygen

Oxygen is our primary life-support. The air we breathe is so vital that without it we would rapidly die. Clean air is made up of several gases of which Oxygen is the most important to us. Clean air contains 19%–21% Oxygen. In ancient times people lived longer because the air was composed of 40% Oxygen. Sadly, the air is decreasing in Oxygen daily.

Every cell in your body requires oxygen every second of the day. Oxygen is your cells' number one nutrient. Proper oxygen delivery cell of your body is absolutely essential, seeing as all of your body functions depend on breathing.

Some experts believe oxygen deficiency is the single greatest cause of all disease. Deep breathing fights off disease in more than one way. Most importantly, it provides your cells with the oxygen they require to function

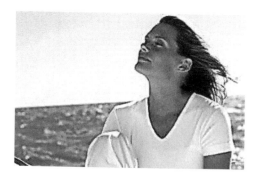

well and stay healthy. In addition, deep breathing, like exercise, helps moves your lymphatic fluid through your body. You actually create a vacuum effect inside you when you take a deep breath, which pulls the lymphatic fluid throughout your immune system. Cancer, infection, and disease of every sort hate oxygen, so fight them off by taking a deep breath of fresh air.

Besides balancing your immune system, deep breathing also enhances detoxification, the other part of the health equation. Deep breathing can increase your body's rate of toxin elimination by as much as fifteen times the normal rate. That's huge!

Most people, even seasoned athletes, breathe well below 100 percent efficiency. In fact, the average person uses considerably less than 25 percent of their actual lung capacity during normal breathing. Granted, the lungs have a tremendous 'reserve' capacity, which is to say that none of us needs to be breathing at, or even near, full capacity to procure all the oxygen we need under normal circumstances. Even so, the more fully you can breathe, the more easily you can oxygenate your many tissues to increase the overall efficiency of your respiratory process.

The human body is largely composed of oxygen, so it is no wonder that scientists are now discovering how low levels of oxygen can disrupt the body's ability to function correctly. The oxygen concentration in a healthy human body is approximately three times that of air. Fortunately, oxygen is the most abundant element on earth comprising nearly 50% of the earth's crust and averaging about 20% of dry air in a non-polluted environment.

Once you notice that you habitually breathe in a shallow fashion you can remedy the situation. Here are some of the benefits deep breathing will do for you:

> • Purifies the bloodstream, allowing a detoxification to take place in the body.

• More efficient digestion due to increased oxygen reaching the stomach.

• Improved health of the brain, spinal cord, and nerves due to increased oxygen.

• Skin becomes smoother and healthier with a reduction in facial wrinkles.

• Healthier more powerful lungs, increasing stamina.

• Rejuvenates glands in the body including pituitary and pineal glands.

• Allows heart to last longer and work more efficiently.

• Fights against heart disease by providing extra oxygen to your heart's tissues.

• Relaxes mind and body without inducing tiredness. You feel relaxed and energized at the same time.

• Releases tension and reduces stress.

All of the above will leave you more energized, full of life, and healthier than before. These are powerful effects from something as simple as deep breathing.

Practice deep, slow breathing as many times as you can throughout the day. Even if you only stop for a second and take two deep breaths it is a start. Here is how you deep breathe properly:

1. Fully exhale all air out of your system, making sure to completely empty the lungs.

2. Breathe in through your nose into your lower abdomen. You want

According to a 3 year study at Harvard University, exposure to bright sunlight first thing will have a positive impact on the retina that leads to better focus and energy production in the brain. For many people, bright sunlight in the morning will improve their mood and increase their alertness.

the lower part of the lungs to fill with air first, then the upper. Fully fill your lungs until they reach their capacity.

3. Slowly exhale all air out through your mouth, being sure to completely empty the lungs.

4. Repeat.

As you can see this is very simple. What you are doing is using your lungs to their complete capacity. This will quickly oxygenate your body and allow for increased strength, energy, and vitality.

The more time you spend deep breathing each day the better your results will be. Why don't you take a deep breath right now and let all of your tensions melt away?

Many people don't know the powerful effects deep breathing has on your health and vitality. It is strange that something as fundamental as breathing goes unnoticed as being a powerful contributing factor to one's health.

Sufficient oxygen helps the body in its ability to rebuild itself and maintain a strong and healthy immune system. Although we know that vitamins, minerals and enzymes are necessary for our health and vitality, you can actually exist without food for about 40 days, and go without water for about seven days. Without oxygen, a crucial life-support, life ceases to exist in only minutes.

Benefits of Sunlight

- One of the major benefits of sunlight is that it helps fruits, vegetables, and grains to grow and be healthy. It also helps animals and us humans to grow and develop as well.
- A definite plus of sunshine is that it gives you a healthy looking complexion. It will make your skin smooth with an irresistible healthy glow.
- If you get regular exposure to sunlight, it will help protect your skin in the long run. That is because your body will build up a natural resistance to the harmful effects of ultraviolet light.
- If you allow your skin to get moderately tanned, it will be more resistant to infections and sunburns than if your skin is not tanned.

- The ultraviolet rays in sunshine act as a natural antiseptic. These rays can kill viruses, bacteria, molds, yeasts, fungi, and mites in air, water, and on different surfaces including your skin.
- Getting some sun tends to help clear up different skin diseases such as acne, boils, athletes foot, diaper rash, psoriasis, and eczema.
- Another of the main benefits of sunlight is that it stimulates your appetite and improves your digestion, elimination, and metabolism.
- Getting your daily dose of sunshine will enhance your immune system. It increases the number of white blood cells in your blood. It also helps them to be better fighters in their mission to destroy germs.
- Sunshine encourages healthy circulation. It also stimulates the production of more red blood cells which increases the amount of oxygen in your blood.
- Sunlight is one of the most effective healing agents that exist.
- Feeling down? One of the major benefits of sunlight is that it will soothe your nerves and boost your mood leaving you with a renewed sense of well-being. Sunlight increases the production of endorphins and serotonin in your brain which will definitely leave you feeling much better.
- Getting enough sunlight during the day can help you sleep better at night. If you are exposed to natural light during the day, it will increase your melatonin output at night. Melatonin is a natural hormone made by our bodies. It enhances sleep and slows down the aging process.
- The healing properties of the sun are excellent for people who are suffering from various diseases and ailments.
- Sunlight helps to balance out your hormones. It may even help to relieve certain symptoms of PMS.
- Sunlight improves the function of your liver and helps it to break down toxins and wastes that could lead to cancer and other diseases.
- If you've got swollen, arthritic joints, sunlight may help lower your pain levels.
- Sunlight is an effective treatment for jaundice.
- According to some studies on the benefits of sunlight, exposure to the sun may decrease your risk of breast, colon, and prostate cancers.

- Sunlight helps your body convert a form of cholesterol that is present in your skin into vitamin D. This results in lower blood cholesterol levels.
- Other benefits of sunlight include the life-giving energy it gives to your organs and the way it helps to strengthen and vitalize your body.

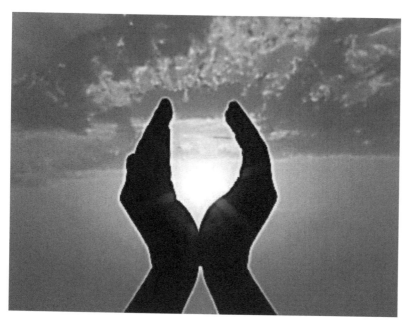

What If I Don't Get Enough Sunlight?

Not getting enough direct sunlight on your skin can have a negative effect on your health. Lack of sunlight can worsen feelings of depression in some people.

According to one study in the American Journal of Clinical Nutrition your chances of getting cancer could increase by as much as 70% if you don't get enough direct sunlight.

If you do not get enough sunlight your body may not make enough vitamin D. Having a vitamin D deficiency may put you at increased risk for bone diseases such as osteoporosis. Low vitamin D levels can also cause weak hearts, poor metabolism, and slow healing of bones and cuts.

Researchers have started recognizing the importance of sunlight for a healthy lifestyle, recent studies reveal that sunlight renders many health benefits. Apart from Sunlight maintaining temperature and humidity, sunlight plays a significant role in nourishing and energizing the human body. It is also vital in order to get the full nutritional value from food that you consume and it has been proven that getting sufficient sunlight aids in preventing chronic ailments such as seasonal affective disorder (SAD), osteoporosis, mental depression, type 2 diabetes, and cancers affecting the bladder, breasts, cervix, colon, ovaries, prostrate, and the stomach. To put it more succinctly, sunlight serves as the perfect medicinal pill in promoting a healthy lifestyle.

For you to feel your best, heal conditions, sleep better, and find your happy self again, you need to breath deeper and find time for sunlight. This chapter is amazing. Never underestimate the power of God's simple creations. The power of breath. The power of sunlight. The power of nature and green plants. The power of the sounds of birds, ocean waves, and bubbling brooks. These all have major healing properties. You are learning some basic ways to heal the body, holistically. It just makes sense. Nature needs no help, it just needs no interference.

Chapter 15

Water - Hydrate for Health

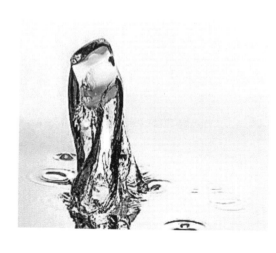

Your body is mostly made up of water. Between 65 and 70 percent is water; your brain is more than 80 percent water, your blood is more than 90 percent water. Since your blood is mostly water and "the life of the flesh is in the blood" (Leviticus 17:11), you need water, water, and more water to be healthy.

You lose approximately 64 ounces of water a day from breathing, urination, and sweating, so you need to drink eight eight-ounces glasses of water just to break even and replenish yourself. Yet few people break even and most people drink much less. I cannot overestimate the number of people who walk around chronically dehydrated! The twelfth step to your BETTER BODY is keeping yourself hydrated.

Do you often get fatigued, irritable, depressed, confused, or upset by intense food cravings? You simply could be dehydrated. You can do a couple easy tests for dehydration. First, lightly pinch the skin on the back of your hand together and pull upward. If your skin doesn't immediately recede back into place when you let go, but rather stays raised for a few seconds, you need more water. Second, check the color of your urine. It should be light, not dark or even yellow. If your urine is colored, you need more water. Dehydration creates a multitude of physical problems.

Water is the ultimate detoxifier. An increase of only five glasses a day may cut the risk of colon cancer by 45%, bladder cancer by 50%, and breast cancer by 79%. Cancer can only develop in an acidic environment, and guess what dehydration does? It causes your body to be acidic. Many of us live right on the edge of acidity—a real risk to our health—but the more water we drink, the more balanced our pH levels will be.

More Water = Less Disease

Your appreciation for water will increase if you'll only start drinking it. Try adding a slice of lemon or lime, or cooling your water in summer and warming it in winter. Leave out the sugary powered drink mixes, hot chocolate, or coffee, though. Those don't have the same good effects on your health as water—quite the opposite. We'll see why shortly. First, here's a simple way to figure out how much water you need every day. Divide your weight in pounds by 2 and drink that many ounces of water. If you weight 150, divide by 2 and drink 74 ounces a day—about 10 cups. That way at least you're replenishing what you're losing, and once you're used to that amount, drink some more!

Water Cure: Healing Your Body through Rehydration

The urgent cries from our body to give it a drink of pure water is by far the most serious signal from the human body to ignore. The 3 trillion cells that make up your body have certain daily requirements. One of the most vital one is water. Water affects every tissue, organ, gland, chemical reaction, nutrient transportation, hormonal communication, healing and repairing the body, electrical stimulation (heart rhythms), and elimination function of the body.

Pure Water

The body needs pure water; not tea, coffee, soda, juice, or milk to maintain the best health status. People have become de-sensitized of the word "water" with "liquids". I ask every patient "how much water do you consume each day?" Nearly each answer is filled with "well I drink 3 cups of coffee and 2 sodas each day, which counts right?" Others say, "Does that does that mean juice and milk?" Our society has been bombarded with media hypes on who's energy "drink" is the best and who's "soda" is the best. Or worse yet, who's "flavored water" are the best? Where did plain water disappear to? Is it coincidence the time all the flavored "liquids" came out that health problems started to come forward?

And people wonder why they have strange rashes coming up, why they can't sleep at night, why their blood pressure is high, why they can't focus or remember things, why their stomach produces too much acid (or not enough), or why they are overweight. It could simply lie in the fact they are dehydrated. It is a catastrophic mistake to overlook the need of water.

Our bodies first started out in water for nine months. We need it to cleanse ourselves, we need it to cook with, we use it for recreation, and we use it to quench our "thirst". Water is very calming to be around. But most importantly, we need it for the physiological events that happen within our bodies. As stated earlier, every cell, tissue, gland, and organ needs it to survive. The brain requires the most amount of water of all organs (30%). Could it be that all the kids that are tagged with ADD and ADHD could just be dehydrated from water.

Dehydration

So if you suffer from: constipation, arthritis, allergies, insomnia, diabetes, tense muscles, high blood pressure, or losing your memory you likely are dehydrated. The number one cause of night time muscle spasms (Charley horses) is chronic dehydration for people over 50. Start drinking 8 glasses or bottles of pure water (not flavored because then you are adding artificial chemicals) a day and see if your conditions start to disappear. It takes about 2 weeks for you to get readjusted to drinking more fluids and to acquire the taste. So if you are urinating more often, that's fine, hang in there. Your urine should be clear to light yellow.

According to Dr. Batmanghelidj, MD, author of <u>Your Body's Many Cries for Water</u>, states that majority of health problems start with the dehydration of pure water factor. He says most medical doctors have forgotten to ask and educate on the premise of proper water consumption. He says "don't treat thirst with medications". Meaning, many people are given medications for conditions that are mainly dehydration issues. "Medical practitioners have been taught to *silence* these signals (simple dehydration) with chemical products." He goes on to add, "The simple truth is dehydration can cause disease".

According to Dr. Michael Colgan, if you dehydrate a muscle by only 3%, you lose 10% contractile strength and 8% of your speed. Staying hydrated is very important to both lifelong health and top physical performance.

One person at a time needs to realize the healthcare crisis is our responsibility. You need to become educated and listen to the basic information being presented on nutrition, diet, exercise, lifestyle, stress management, and proper hydration. Because once you start knowing how your body works, and what makes it start falling apart, you can prevent it! This will save the economy billions of dollars in healthcare.

Do not assume that eating fast food, drinking soda, not exercising, not dealing with stress will affect you, because it will, it is like a time bomb, just waiting to go off. Will you control your fate, or will fate control you?

Start with some simple changes. Buy bottled water instead of soda. Use a filtration system for your home tap water. Have a monthly water cooler installed in your home. Ask about home filtration systems. Use the simple math for how much to drink each day (drink ½ your body weight in ounces per day).

Drinking water is a vital piece to achieving health, wellness, and longevity. If you consume your daily requirements of water you may gain quality years to your life. You will feel better, look better, function better and may even be able to get off some medications just by re-hydrating your body. Water is free many times, widely available, and always a choice to choose from. Start with drinking more water for your health. Treat your Temple with the power of hydration.

Healthy Homemade Recipes

Breakfast

Blueberry-Cucumber Smoothie

Blended cucumbers thicken a lightly sweet smoothie for a low-calorie breakfast or a refreshing afternoon snack.

> 2 large garden cucumbers, peeled, seeded, and cut into chunks (2 cups)
> 1 cup low-fat vanilla yogurt
> 1 cup frozen blueberries
> 1–2 Tbs. honey or agave nectar
> 1 Tbs. lemon juice

Place all ingredients in blender, and blend until smooth.

Blackberry Banana Breakfast Cake

Ingredients

1 c. almond flour
1/2 c. shredded unsweetened coconut
1 tsp. cinnamon
1 tsp. baking powder
1/2 tsp. baking soda
1/2 tsp. salt
1/4 c. Stevia
1 ripe banana,
2 eggs
1 tsp. vanilla extract
1/2 c. vanilla almond milk
1 c. fresh or frozen
blackberries.

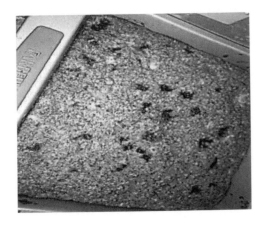

Blend and bake at 350 for 30-35 minutes.

PBJ Protein Oats

Ingredients

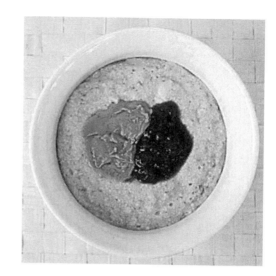

1/3 cup old-fashioned oats
2/3 cup water
1 serving vanilla protein powder
1/2 teaspoon vanilla bean paste or extract
1 tablespoon natural peanut butter
1 tablespoon natural jam or jelly

Directions

1. Combine oats and water in a small saucepan and bring to a boil.
2. Reduce heat and let oatmeal simmer until 90% of the water is absorbed.
3. Remove from heat and whisk in protein powder and vanilla.
4. Pour oatmeal into a bowl and top with peanut butter and jelly/jam.

Note: you can also add flax seeds to this

Egg-White Muffin Melt

Ingredients

3 egg whites
Whole-grain English muffin
1/2 cup spinach
1 slice reduced-fat cheddar cheese
1 slice tomato

Make It

Scramble 3 egg whites. Cover half of a whole-grain English muffin with 1/2 cup spinach and the other half with 1 slice reduced-fat cheddar cheese; toast until cheese is melted. Add egg and 1 slice tomato.

Lunch

Grilled Cilantro-Jalapeno Portobello Mushrooms

Ingredients:
3-4 portabella mushroom caps
1 generous handful of cilantro, chopped
3-4 small garlic cloves, chopped or minced
½ jalapeno pepper, chopped
1 green onion, chopped
¼ cup olive oil
1 tbsp. butter
sea salt to taste

Directions:
1. Combine above ingredients.
2. Pour mixture over portabellas and marinate for 30 minutes.
3. Grill or bake mushrooms at 400° F for 8-10 minutes.
4. Serve over quinoa or brown rice.
(Serves 2-4)

Asparagus Salad

Ingredients

8 asparagus spears	2 teaspoons olive oil
1 garlic clove	2 cups mixed greens
1 hard-boiled egg	1 tablespoon vinegar
Salt	
Pepper	

Directions

Cut 8 asparagus spears into 2-inch pieces; sauté with 2 teaspoons olive oil and 1 minced garlic clove. Top 2 cups greens with cooked asparagus, 1 chopped hard-boiled egg, 1 tablespoon vinegar and salt and pepper to taste.

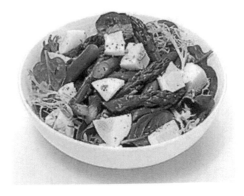

Cool Cucumber and Avocado Soup

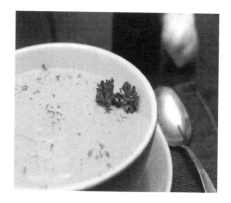

Ingredients:
1 cucumber, peeled and chopped
1 avocado
2 green onions
Juice of 1 lime
1 cup plain Greek yogurt
1 cup water
Salt and pepper to taste

Directions:
1. Roughly chop the cucumber, avocado and green onions and toss in the blender.
2. Add other ingredients and process until smooth.
3. If soup is too thick add water as needed.

Avocado Pesto Pasta

Ingredients:
1 lb. thin rice noodles or buckwheat noodles
1 bunch basil leaves
½ cup walnuts or macadamia nuts
2 ripe avocados, pitted and peeled
2 tablespoons fresh lemon juice
3 cloves fresh garlic, chopped
½ cup olive oil
Salt to taste
Freshly ground black pepper to taste
Rice Grated Topping Parmesan Flavor (optional)

Directions:
1. In a large pot, bring water to a boil. Add pasta and cook to package directions.
2. While pasta cooks, in a food processor, blend basil, nuts, avocados, lemon juice, garlic, and olive oil. Season with salt and pepper.
3. Drain pasta. In a large serving bowl, evenly toss pesto with cooked pasta and serve.
4. For a healthy option instead of dairy cheese, top pasta with Rice Grated Topping parmesan vegan cheese if desired.

Dinner

Baked Cilantro Salmon

Ingredients:
3 10 oz. filets of salmon
6 cloves garlic, sliced
5 tsp. cilantro
2 tsp. honey
juice of one lemon

Directions:
1. Wash and prepare salmon. Set in oven-safe baking dish (foil-lined for ease of clean-up), skin side down.
2. In a small sauté pan, sauté garlic, lemon juice, honey and cilantro over medium to medium-low heat. Let mixture sauté for approximately 5-6 minutes, until heated thoroughly. Remember to mix at regular intervals so that the honey does not caramelize/crystallize onto the pan. Remove from heat and let cool.
3. When the mixture has cooled, spread it evenly over each filet of salmon. Refrigerate salmon and let marinate for up to 30 minutes in the refrigerator.

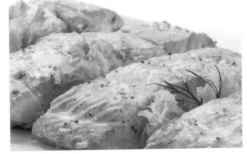

4. Preheat oven to 400° F. Bake salmon for 20 minutes, remove from heat. Let it sit for approximately five minutes before serving.
(Serves 4-6

Zucchini and Potato Bake

Ingredients

2 medium zucchini, quartered and cut into large pieces
4 medium potatoes, peeled and cut into large chunks
1 medium red bell pepper, seeded and chopped
1 clove garlic, sliced   1/2 cup dry bread crumbs
1/4 cup olive oil   paprika to taste
salt to taste   ground black pepper to taste

Directions

Preheat oven to 400 degrees F (200 degrees C).

In a medium baking pan, toss together the zucchini, potatoes, red bell pepper, garlic, bread crumbs, and olive oil. Season with paprika, salt, and pepper.

Bake 1 hour in the preheated oven, stirring occasionally, until potatoes are tender and lightly brown.

Zucchini With Quinoa Stuffing

Ingredients

1/2 cup quinoa, rinsed
4 medium zucchini
1 15-ounce can cannellini beans, rinsed
1 cup grape or cherry tomatoes, quartered
1/2 cup almonds, chopped (about 2 ounces)
2 cloves garlic, chopped
3/4 cup grated Parmesan (3 ounces)
4 tablespoons olive oil

Directions

1. Heat oven to 400° F. In a large saucepan, combine the quinoa and 1 cup water and bring to a boil. Reduce heat to medium-low, cover, and simmer until the quinoa is tender and the water is absorbed, 12 to 15 minutes.

2. Meanwhile, cut the zucchini in half lengthwise and scoop out the seeds. Arrange in a large baking dish, cut-side up.

3. Fluff the quinoa and fold in the beans, tomatoes, almonds, garlic, ½ cup of the Parmesan, and 3 tablespoons of the oil.

4. Spoon the mixture into the zucchini. Top with the remaining tablespoon of oil and ¼ cup Parmesan. Cover with foil and bake until the zucchini is tender, 25 to 30 minutes. Remove the foil and bake until golden, 8 to 10 minutes.

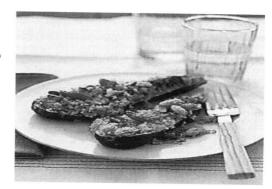

Lemon-Thyme Chicken with Sautéed Vegetables

Ingredients:

4 tablespoons lemon juice
1 tablespoon chopped garlic, divided
1 tablespoon chopped fresh thyme, divided
1 pound chicken breast tenders, lightly pounded
1 1/2 cups frozen shelled edamame, thawed
11/2 cups grape tomatoes, halved
2 medium zucchini   1/3 cup crumbled feta
4 teaspoons canola oil   1 medium shallot, sliced
Salt   Freshly ground black pepper

Directions:

1. In a zip lock bag, combine 3 tablespoons lemon juice, 2 teaspoons garlic, and 2 teaspoons thyme; season to taste with salt and black pepper. Add chicken tenders, seal the bag, and gently turn to coat. Set aside.
2. Heat 2 teaspoons canola oil in a large skillet over medium-high heat. Add shallot, remaining garlic, edamame, and tomatoes; sauté 4 minutes.
3. Use a vegetable peeler to slice zucchini into long ribbons. Add zucchini and remaining lemon juice and thyme to vegetables in skillet; sauté 2 to 3 minutes. Transfer to a serving bowl, stir in feta, and season with salt and black pepper to taste.
4. Add remaining oil to skillet. Remove chicken from marinade and sauté 2 to 3 minutes a side or until cooked through. Serve with vegetables.

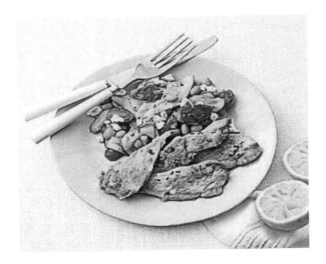

Snacks

No Bake Energy Bites (YUMMY ☺)

Ingredients:

1 cup oatmeal

1/3 cup honey

1/2 cup ground flaxseed

1 tsp. vanilla

1/2 cup peanut butter (or other nut butter)

1 cup coconut flakes

1/2 cup mini chocolate chips

Directions

Mix together and roll into balls. Store in a sealed container in the fridge.

Baked Banana Oatmeal Cups

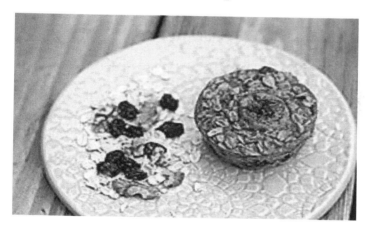

Ingredients

2 cups old fashioned oatmeal

1/2 teaspoon sea salt

1/3 cup egg whites

1 teaspoon organic vanilla extract

1 Tablespoon coconut oil, in liquid form

6 drops liquid stevia OR 1packet of powdered stevia OR 1/3 cup maple syrup

2 cups unsweetened vanilla almond milk

1/4 cup walnuts OR almonds OR other nut

2 teaspoons ground cinnamon

1 teaspoon baking powder

2 medium bananas, mashed

1/2-3/4 cup raisins

Directions

Preheat oven to 350 degrees and spray one 12-cup muffin pan with cooking spray or line with cupcake liners.

In a bowl mix together oatmeal, cinnamon, sea salt and baking powder.

In another bowl mix together egg whites, coconut oil, vanilla, stevia and mashed bananas until combined. Dump dry ingredients into wet ingredients; mix well. Pour in almond milk and stir until combined.

Gently stir in walnuts and raisins. Scoop the mixture evenly into muffin cups.

Bake 30-35 minutes or until the center of each oatmeal cup is set and a toothpick comes out clean.

Baked Bananas

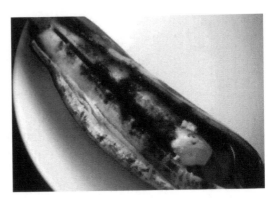

Ingredients

4 firm bananas
1 tsp. olive oil
1-inch piece grated fresh ginger
1 tbsp. cinnamon
1/2 tbsp. nutmeg
1/2 cup raisins

Directions

Preheat oven to 375 degrees.
Peel and cut bananas in half, lengthwise.
Oil a baking pan and arrange bananas.
Sprinkle with cinnamon, nutmeg, ginger and raisins.
Cover and bake for 10 to 15 minutes.

Note: This is wonderful with chocolate sauce!

Watermelon Salsa

Ingredients

3 cups finely diced seedless watermelon, (about 2 1/4 pounds with the rind) (see Tip)
2 jalapeno peppers, seeded and minced (see Ingredient note)
1/3 cup chopped cilantro, (about 1/2 bunch)
1/4 cup lime juice
1/4 cup minced red onion, (about 1/2 small)
1/4 teaspoon salt, or to taste

Directions

1. Place watermelon, jalapenos, cilantro, lime juice and onion in a medium bowl; stir well to combine. Season with salt. Serve at room temperature or chilled.

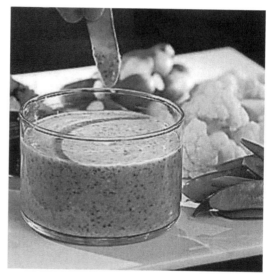

Feta & Herb Dip

Ingredients

1 15-ounce can white beans, rinsed   3/4 cup nonfat plain yogurt
1/2 cup crumbled feta cheese
1 teaspoon freshly ground pepper
1/4 cup chopped fresh parsley
1/4 cup chopped fresh mint

1 tablespoon lemon juice
1 teaspoon garlic salt
1/4 cup chopped fresh dill
1/4 cup chopped fresh chives

Directions

Place beans, yogurt, feta, lemon juice, garlic salt and pepper in a food processor and puree until smooth. Add herbs; puree until incorporated. Chill until ready to serve. Serve with assorted vegetables, such as baby carrots, bell pepper strips, radishes, snow peas, broccoli and cauliflower florets.
MAKE AHEAD TIP: Cover and refrigerate for up to 2 days.

References and Resources

Ansari Ph. D., Moin S. *Practical Nutrition: A Nutrition Course Workbook*. Brady Press, Inc., 1999.

Auer M.D., Wolfgang R. *The Acid Danger: Combating Acidosis Correctly*. Laguna Beach, CA: Basic Health Publication, Inc., 2004.

Balch CNC, Phyllis and James F. Balch, M.D.. *Prescription for Nutritional Healing*. New York, NY:
Avery Publishing, 2000, 3rd Edition.

Barbee C.D.C., Michael. *Politically Incorrect Nutrition*. Ridgefield, CT: Vital Health Publishing, 2004.

Baroody M.D., Theodore A. *Alkalize or Die*. Waynesville, NC: Holographic Health Press, 1991.

Batmanghelidj MD, F. *Your Body's Many Cries for Water*. Falls Church, VA: Global Health Solutions, Inc., 1995.

Berkson, D. Lindsey. *Hormone Deception*. Chicago, IL :Contemporary Publishing, 2001.

Bernstein, M.D., Richard K. *The Diabetes Diet*. New York, NY: Little, Brown and Company, 2005.

Centers for Disease Control and Prevention. *Rising Health Care Costs Are Unsustainable*. April 2011.

Centers for Medicare and Medicaid Services, Office of the Actuary, National Health Statistics Group, *National Health Care Expenditures Data*, January 2012.

Colbert MD, Don. *Living in Divine Health*. Lake Mary, FL: Siloam, 2006.

Colbert MD, Don. *The Bible Cure for Weight Loss & Muscle Gain*. Lake Mary, FL: Siloam, 2000.

Colbert MD, Don. *Toxic Relief*. Lake Mary, FL: Siloam, 2001.

Congress of the United States, Congressional Budget Office. *Technological Change and the Growth of Health Care Spending*, January 2008.

Cook DNM, DAc, Michelle S. *The Ultimate pH Solution*. New York, NY: HarpersCollins Publishers, 2008.

Elkins M.H., Rita. *Digestive Enzymes*. Pleasant Grove, UT: Woodland Publishing, 1998.

Hofmekler, Ori. *The Anti-Estrogenic Diet*. Berkley, CA: North Atlantic Books, 2007

Jackson Ph.D., Nisha. The Hormone Survival Guide for Perimenopause. Santa Rosa, CA: Larkfield Publishing, 2004.

Leaf M.D., Caroline. Who Switched Off My Brain? Controlling Toxic Thoughts and Emotions. United States of America: Switch On Your Brain, 2007.

Lipton Ph.D., Bruce H. *Biology of Belief.* United States of America: Mountain of Love Productions, 2008.

Lipton Ph.D., Bruce H. The Wisdom of Your Cells: How Your Beliefs Control Your Biology. 2006 CD.

Martin, A.B. et al. January 2012. *Growth in US health spending remained slow in 2010; Health share of gross domestic product was unchanged from 2009.* Health Affairs 31(1): 208-219.

Mead M.D., Jay H. and Erin T. Lommen, N.D. *Slim Sane & Sexy: Pocket Guide to Natural, Bioidentical Hormone Balancing.* Rancho Mirage, CA: Fountain of Youth Press, 2008.

Peale, Norman Vincent. The Power of Positive Thinking. New York, NY: Simon & Schuster, 2003

Pilzer, Paul Zane. The Wellness Revolution: How to Make a Fortune in the Next Trillion Dollar Industry. New York: NY: John Wiley & Sons Inc., 2002

Reid, Daniel. *The Complete Book of Chinese Health & Healing.* Boston, MA: Shambhala Publishing, Inc., 1994.

Richards, Byron J. *Fight for Your Health: Exposing the FDA's Betrayal of America.* Tucson, AZ: Truth in Wellness, LLC., 2006.

Smith M.D., Pamela Wartian. *Why You Can't Lose Weight: Why it's so Hard to Shed Pounds and What You Can Do About It.* Garden City Park, NY: Square One Publishers, 2011.

Trudeau, Kevin. *The Weight Loss Cure.* Elk Grove, IL: Alliance Publishing Group, Inc., 2007.

Vasey N.D., Christopher. The Acid-Alkaline Diet for Optimum Health. Rochester, VT: Healing Arts Press, 1999.

VerHulst M.D., Don. *10 Keys That Cure – Bible Truths for Better Health Today.* United States of America: Don VerHulst M.D., 2008.

Wilson N.D., D.C., Ph.D., James, L. *Adrenal Fatigue: The 21st Century Stress Syndrome.* Petaluma, CA: Smart Publications, 2003.

Yost, Graham. *Vitamins and Minerals.* Springhouse, PA: Springhouse Corporation, 1986.

Young Ph.D., Robert O., and Shelley Redford Young. *The pH Miracle: Balance Your Diet, Reclaim Your Health.* New York, NY: Wellness Central, 2002.

Websites

Hyman MD, Mark. *Is Your Body Burning Up With Hidden Inflammation?* (accessed 09/08/2012) http://drhyman.com/blog/conditions/is-your-body-burning-up-with-hidden-inflammation/

INFORMATION RESOURCES INC , *Consumer and Shopper Insights Advantage.* (accessed 10/02/2012) http://www.symphonyiri.com/LinkClick.aspx?fileticket=lMxgJc0cxCY=&t abid=348

Kresser L.AC., Chris. 9 Steps to Perfect Health-#5: Heal Your Gut. (accessed 09/08/2012) http://chriskresser.com/9-steps-to-perfect-health-5-heal-your-gut

Levi PhD, Jeffrey. *Most Americans May Be Obese by 2030, Report Warns.* (accessed 09/21/2012) http://abcnews.go.com/Health/americans-obese-2030-report-warns/story?id=17260134#.UHIEScA8CSo

Lee MD, John. *Saliva Hormone Testing.* (accessed 09/15/2012) http://www.johnleemd.com/store/saliva_serum.html

Organization for Economic Co-Operation and Development (OECD). *Heath Statistics* (accessed 09/02/2012) http://stats.oecd.org/index.aspx?DataSetCode=HEALTH_STAT

Pick, Dr. Marcelle, OB/GYN. *Phytotherapy — the key to hormonal balance?* (accessed 12/30/2011) http://www.womentowomen.com/menopause/phytotherapy.aspx

Rice, Sabriya. Are you taking too many meds? (accessed 08/25/2012) http://www.cnn.com/2011/HEALTH/05/31/med.nation.too.many.meds/index.html

Toppo, Greg. Study: Senior's Drug Costs Soar. (accessed 9/20/2012) http://abcnews.go.com/Health/story?id=118104&page=1#.UG5M9MA8CSo

Webb D.C., Charles. *Hormone Health: How to Get Your Hormones Back in Balance* (accessed 9/15/2012)http://drcharleswebb.com/Hormones.pdf

Zenhabits. *20 Ways to Eliminate Stress from Your Life* (accessed 09/15/2012) http://zenhabits.net/20-ways-to-eliminate-stress-from-your-life/

Zwillich, Todd. *Drugs for Seniors: A Costly Problem* (accessed 9/16/2012) http://www.medicinenet.com/script/main/art.asp?articlekey=50439

Resources

Angie Cross, D.C.
Healing Arts Center
715 N. Clark St.
Carroll, IA 51401   phone: 712-792-4600
Email: angiecrossdc@yahoo.com
www.carrollhealingarts.com
www.drangiecross.com

www.yoli.com

www.yoli.com/gettingstarted

www.brimhallwellness.com

www.nutriwest.com

www.labrix.com

www.neuroscienceinc.com

www.palmer.edu

Stephanie Fisher, CHC
Nutritional Performance and Wellness
330 W. 3rd Street
Glidden, IA 51443   phone: 712-830-6170
Email: nutritionalperformance@gmail.com
www.mynutritionalperformance.com

www.antiestrogenicdiet.com

www.womenlivingnaturally.com

www.south-beach-diet-plan.com

www.womentowomen.com

www.hormone.org

www.johnleemd.com

www.menopause.org

www.naturalbiohealth.com

www.yourphlife.com

www.phbodybalance.com

www.balancephforlife.com

INDEX

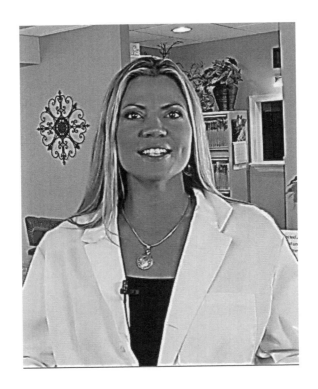

ABOUT THE AUTHOR

Dr. Angie Cross is a 2003 graduate of Palmer College of Chiropractic. She is passionate about chiropractic and natural holistic options to treat the body and mind. She has spent the last 15 years studying and learning everything she can find about natural and holistic healing avenues. She has been trained extensively in the 6 Steps to Wellness™ by the Brimhall technique. She runs and operates The Healing Arts Center in Carroll, Iowa. She uses acupuncture, herbal therapies, detoxification programs, saliva testing with bio-identical hormone replacements, emotional releasing techniques, low level therapy, and specific diet recommendations. She is a speaker on the topics of chiropractic, holistic health, hormonal balancing, and natural weight loss. In addition to her private practice, she offers personalized online individual and group coaching, testing and health resources. DrAngieCross.com also offers products and solutions to help people reach their goals. Her primary interest is working with middle aged women who struggle with hormonal and weight issues.

Made in the USA
San Bernardino, CA
20 November 2013